Friedrich Kummer (ed.)

Treatment of Asthma: The long-acting beta-2-agonists

SpringerWienNewYork

Prof. Dr. med. Friedrich Kummer
2. Medizinische Abteilung mit Lungenkrankheiten und Tuberkulose,
Wilhelminenspital, Wien, Österreich

Typesetting: H. Meszarics • Satz & Layout • A-1200 Wien

Graphic design: Ecke Bonk

Printed on acid-free and chlorine-free bleached paper
SPIN: 10675873

With 35 Figures

Library of Congress Cataloging-in-Publication Data

Treatment of asthma : the long-acting beta-2-agonists / Friedrich Kummer (Hrsg.)
p.cm.
Includes bibliographical references and index.
ISBN-13:978-3-211-83124-3 e-ISBN-13:978-3-7091-7513-2
DOI: 10.1007/978-3-7091-7513-2

1. Asthma – Chemotherapy. 2. Adrenergic beta agonists.
I. Kummer, Friedrich.
[DNLM: 1. Asthma – drug therapy. 2. Adrenergic beta-Agonists – therapeutic use.
3. Adrenergic beta-Agonists – pharmacology. WF 553 T784 1998]
RC591.T74 1998
616.2'38061 – dc21

ISBN-13:978-3-211-83124-3

Preface

The traditional Vienna Asthma Forum was held in early June 1996 and was the 6th in a biennial mode within 10 years.

This time it was dedicated to the long-acting beta-2-agonists, which were registered (or just about to be) in most European countries.

The introduction of this therapeutic principle into routine praxis of asthma therapy was so successful that a closer view on the subject from a scientific point was warranted. Salmeterol, shortly afterwards formoterol are the drugs available for the inhalative route, while bambuterol serves as an oral agent.

The scientists particularly involved in the design and pharmacokinetics of these drugs were invited, and we were lucky that Malcolm Johnson (Glaxo), Leif Svensson (Astra) and Gary Anderson (Ciba-Geigy) delivered fascinating contributions.

However, drug therapy of this kind can only be effective if based on a thorough understanding of the molecular biology of cells and receptors, which was superbly covered by Sheila Collins (Durham) and Ian M. Adcock (London).

The pediatric indications for beta-2-agonists were commented by Manfred Götz (Vienna), and a large spectrum of clinical studies, reported by G. Boyd (Glasgow), A.P. Greening (Edinburgh), M. Rudolph (Middlesex), O. Selroos (Lund) and B. Villiger (Davos) evoked the mutual acid interest of speakers and audience, who engaged in vivid, high quality discussions. The clinical round up and outlook to the future was contributed by Leo Fabbri (Ferrara), who – as an important representative of the European School of Respiratory Medicine – gave the touch of the European Respiratory Society to the entire meeting.

We were keen to include the complete discussion into the proceedings mediating the lively spirit and intense interest of all participants.

Vienna, May 1998 *Univ.-Prof. Dr. F. Kummer*

Contents

Contributors IX

Collins, S., Wang, S.: Molecular regulation of the β_2-adrenergic receptor by long- and short-acting β-agonists 1

Adcock, I.M., Stevens, D.A.: Molecular interactions between glucocorticoids and β_2-agonists 15

Anderson, G.: Formoterol, a new long-acting β_2-agonist 41

Johnson, M.: Development of the long-acting β_2-agonist, salmeterol 43

Svensson, L.-Å.: Development of bambuterol; a long acting, orally active beta-agonist prodrug 71

Götz, M.: Development of β_2-receptors in infancy and childhood 91

Villiger, B.: Long-acting beta-agonists in exercise induced asthma 109

Boyd, G.: Salmeterol and oral steroid treatment 113

Greening, A.P.: Salmeterol and its relationship to treatment with inhaled corticosteroids 121

Rudolf, M.: Long term treatment with formoterol 139

Selroos, O.: Comparison of efficiency of bambuterol and salmeterol 155

Papi, A., Beghé, B., Caramori, G., Ciaccia, A, Fabbri, L.M.: The future of relievers and controllers in asthma therapy 165

Contributors

Dr. Ian M. Adcock, Department of Thoracic Medicine, Imperial College School of Medicine at NHLI, London, U. K.

Dr. Gary Anderson, Department of Pharmacology, University of Melbourne, Australia

Dr. Gavin Boyd, Consultant Respiratory Physician, Stobhill Hospital, Glasgow, U.K.

Dr. Sheila Collins, Duke University Medical Center, Division of Biological Psychiatry and Pharmacology, S.W. Stedman Center for Nutritional Studies, Durham, North Carolina, U.S.A.

Alberto Papi, Laboratorio di Ricerca sull'Asma Bronchiale, Azienda Ospedaliera S. Anna, 3° Piano Nuove Cliniche, Ferrara, Italy

Manfred Götz, M.D., Professor of Paediatrics, Head, Department of Paediatric and Adolescent Medicine, Wilhelminenspital, Vienna, Austria

Dr. Andrew Greening, Consultant Physician, Respiratory Medicine Clinic, Western General Hospital, Edinburgh, U. K.

Dr. Malcolm Johnson, Glaxo Wellcome Research & Development, Uxbridge, Middlesex, U.K.

Dr. Michael Rudolf, Department of Respiratory Medicine, Ealing Hospital, Southall Middlesex, U.K.

Prof. Dr. Olof Selroos, Lund, Sweden

Prof. Dr. Leif-Ake Svensson, Department of Medicinal Chemistry, Astra Draco AB, Lund, Sweden

Dr. Beat Villiger, Swiss Olympic Medical Center, Sportmed SO, Davos Platz, Switzerland

Molecular regulation of the β_2-adrenergic receptor by long- and short-acting β-agonists

S. Collins and *S. Wang*

Duke University Medical Center, Durham, North Carolina, U.S.A.

Summary

Prolonged exposure to β-agonists significantly decreases β-adrenergic receptor (βAR)-stimulated adenylyl cyclase activity and receptor number in a variety of tissues or cells, including the airway. This phenomena is referred to a desensitization, and includes both short-term receptor uncoupling from G proteins and longer term receptor down-regulation. Salmeterol, a new β_2AR-selective agonist, is widely used as one of the most effective, long-acting bronchodilators for the treatment of nocturnal asthma. Interestingly, it can remain efficacious for as long as 12 hours without promoting functional desensitization. Despite its unique characteristics of resistance to desensitization, the effect of salmeterol on the β_2AR-adenylyl cyclase system has not been fully understood. We have previously demonstrated that the β_2AR gene can be transcriptionally regulated by its own second messenger, cAMP, through the binding and activation of cAMP response element binding protein (CREB). The present study attempted to explore the molecular regulation of the β_2AR by salmeterol in comparison with the shorter-acting βAR-agonist isoproterenol in human bronchial epithelial BEAS-2B cells, a cell line which has been widely used as a model for understanding the regulation of β_2AR in the human airway. Our results demonstrates that brief stimulation (10 min) of cells with 10 nM salmeterol produced a modest, but persistant, stimulation of intracellular cAMP levels over several hours. Moreover, during a period of chronic exposure, salmeterol-treated cells do not display the down-regulation of β_2AR mRNA levels as observed in isoproterenol-treated cells. Thus, this differential effect on salmeterol on β_2AR gene expression may contribute to the ability of this agonist to sustain β_2AR-mediated responsiveness, maintaining β_2AR number and functional signal transduction. We present a working model to interpret these results.

Introduction

The β_2AR is one of the G protein-coupled transmembrane receptors that mediate actions of a variety of agents including hormones, neurotransmitters, and even odors and light. A basic scheme for this system is shown in Fig. 1. In the case of the β_2AR, following stimulation with

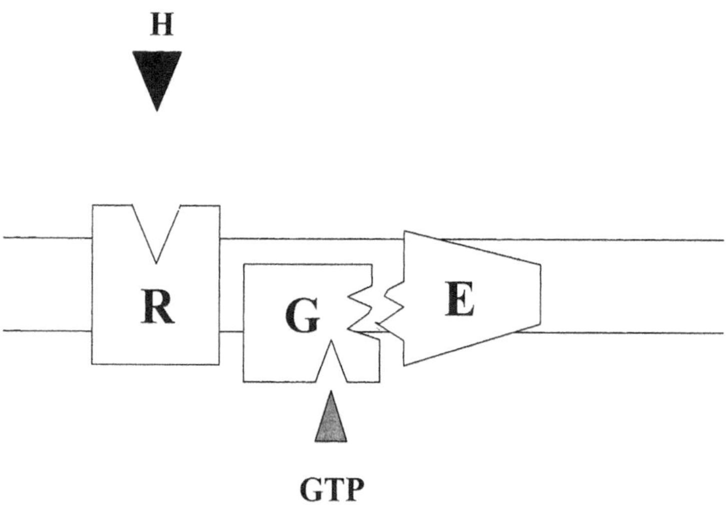

Fig. 1. The schematic illustration of the β-adrenergic receptor signaling complex in the plasma membrane. *H* hormone; *R* receptor; *G* G-protein; *E* effector enzyme (e.g. adenylyl cyclase, phospholipase C)

β-agonists the receptor interacts with the "stimulatory" G protein, Gs, to activate adenylyl cyclase and increase the intracellular level of cAMP. Cyclic AMP, in turn, activates the cAMP-dependent protein kinase (PKA). This cascade of events leads to changes in the state of protein phosphorilation as well as in the transcription of particular target genes in a cell, ultimately leading to specific cellular responses. On the other hand, β-agonists also lead to an inhibition of receptor function due, in part, to phosphorylation of the receptor itself by both PKA and receptor-specific kinases.

β_2-adrenergic receptor

The β_2AR gene was the first of the G protein-coupled receptors to be clonded [1]. The deduced structure of the β_2AR is similar to that of the G protein-coupled receptor family in which the receptor consists of seven transmembrane domains [2].

G protein

The G protein is a heterotrimeric complex consisting three subunits, α, β, and γ. The α subunit is distinct for each G protein, and associates with β and γ that are tightly bound to each other as "βγ". An isoprenoid moiety (i.e. a member of a class of unsaturated lipids) covalently modifies the γ subunit, thereby facilitating association of the αβγ complex with the plasma membrane. Upon binding of agonists to a G protein-coupled receptor, the heterotrimeric G protein is activated. The receptor-activated G protein leads to guanosine triphosphate (GTP) replacing guanosine diphosphate (GDP) on the α subunit, and causing the dissociation of the α from the βγ subunits. The α subunit is then able to activate an effector, transducing the signals further "down the road". During the last few years, the βγ complex has also been found to perform important signal transduction functions [3, 4].

Desensitization

Activation of receptors by agonists, and transduction of the signal to the effector, is frequently followed by a period of refrectoriness or "desensitization". The process of desensitization is a rather general biological phenomenon characterized by a reduction in effector stimulation over time, despite the continuous presence of the stimulus. Desensitization consists of two temporally distinct phenomena: short-term receptor uncoupling [5], and a longer-term receptor down-regulation [6]. Uncoupling is a rapid and reversible process, that uncouples the receptor from Gs within seconds to minutes. Although the ability to generate a response is reduced, the receptor number appears to be unchanged. Moreover, if the agonist is removed, the response can be quickly recovered. The details of this process have been reviewed extensively [5–7].

By contrast, down-regulation requires persistent exposure to the agonist, perhaps minutes to hours depending upon the particular cell type, and results in a dramatic and irreversible reduction in the apparent density of receptors within a cell (Fig. 2). In this case, the recovery can take several hours following removal of the agonist. Invariably new protein synthesis is required, indicating some alteration in the expression of the receptor gene.

1. Uncoupling

Following β_2AR activation, receptor uncoupling is rapidly induced by phosphorylation on cytoplasmic residues of the receptor [1,5,7]. This is certainly one of the major mechanismus by which receptor-mediated signaling is regulated in many systems. Both the cAMP-dependent PKA

Desensitization

Uncoupling	Down-Regulation
rapid	gradual
receptor number unchanged	significant loss of receptors
phosphorylation	irreversible (requires new synthesis)
reversible	altered receptor expression

Fig. 2. Characteristics of agonist-mediated regulation of the β_2-adrenergic receptor

and a receptor-specific kinase ("βARK", more recently termed GRK2 for G-protein-coupled receptor kinase-2) contribute to this alteration in the efficiency of receptor interaction with Gs. In the case of β_2AR, activation of adenylyl cyclase results in generation of cAMP that leads, in turn, to stimulation of PKA catalysis. In addition to other specific intracellular targets, activated PKA phosphorylates amino acid residues in the third cytoplasmic loop and the proximal portion of the carboxyl-terminal tail of β_2AR. As a result, this phosphorylation impairs the coupling of receptor to Gs, interrupting the action of β-agonist.

The GRK2 enzyme displays a more unique, selective phosphorylation of the β_2AR. It phosphorylates only the agonist-occupied, "activated" form of the β_2AR at sites in the serine- and threonine-rich carboxyl terminus. This enzyme shares the basic properties of rhodopsin kinase, an analogous enzyme known to selectively phosphorylate light-activated rhodopsin. This phosphorylation reduces the ability of the receptor to couple to Gs and to activate its effector, adenylyl cyclase. Similar to rhodopsin kinase (also termed GRK1), when GRK2 phosphorylates its receptor substrate, β_2AR, this triggers the recruitment of an additional protein factor called β-arrestin, ("arrestin" in the rhodopsin system) to uncouple and thereby inhibit receptor interaction with Gs [6].

In both the adrenergic receptor and rhodopsin receptor systems, receptor activation is accompanied by translocation of the specific receptor kinases to the plasma membrane. GRK1 is prenylated, thus facilitating its translocation [8]. By contrast, GRK2 is not prenylated. Rather, the translocation of GRK2 to the β_2AR appears to be due to its "delivery" to the receptor by prenylated βγ subunits, following the release of α subunit of Gs protein by receptor activation [3,4].

While it is still not completely clear at the biochemical level how the process of uncoupling is reserved, there is substantial evidence that the rapid and reversible nature of uncoupling is controlled by specific dephosphorylation events. However, many questions remain to be answered about the nature and activity of such phosphatases; including what type(s) of phosphatases, where they are located, and wether there are specific intracellular compartements where receptor dephosphorylation takes place.

2. Down-regulation

There are several distinct processes that participate in the development of down-regulation [6]. These include turnover of the receptor protein and changes in receptor gene trancription. Both cAMP-dependent and -independent mechanisms appear to contribute to down-regulation, with distinct, yet interrelated, effects on both the receptor protein and receptor gene expression [6].

The process of down-regulation of G protein-coupled receptors has been most extensively studied for the β_2AR [6]. Following prolonged exposure with adrenaline over a 24-hours period, there is an approximate 80% decline in receptor number and about 50% decrease in receptor mRNA levels. Consequently, there is a dramatic decrease of the adenylyl cyclase response to β-agonists [9,10]. Several lines of evidence have lead to the notion that receptor down-regulation includes several distinct phenomena. These include:

i) Receptor degradation: The characterization of this pathway has been aided by the use of mutant cell lines defective in either receptor/G protein coupling, adenylyl cyclase stimulation or activation of PKA. Proteolytic degradation of the β_2AR and other G protein-coupled receptors is thougt to contribute significantly to down-regulation, because recovery of a full complement of receptor binding sites has been shown, in most cases, to be a slow process and to require new protein synthesis. However, in most cases this fact has not been unequivocally shown to be true at the biochemical level.

ii) mRNA destabilization: It has been proposes that cAMP-dependent destabilization of β_2AR mRNA leads to a lowered steady-state mRNA levels during down-regulation [9]. An interesting observation related to this issue is that the mRNAs of several G protein-coupled receptors are relatively short-lived. For example, estimated half-life for the β_2AR and D_1-dopamine receptor mRNA ranges from 40 minutes to 1–2 hours [11]. Similarly, for another G protein-coupled receptor, the substance P receptor, that half-life of its mRNA was reported to be about 30 min [12]. Consequently, rapid turnover of receptor mRNAs may provide an additional mechanism, separate from any effects on the receptor protein, for dynamically controlling receptor number and function. In this model, the cell can quickly up- and downregulate the receptor concentration in response to changes in the transcription rate of the receptor. In some cases, down-regulation of the β_2AR has been associated with increased degradation of the receptor mRNA [9]. However, altered mRNA stability may not be a general mechanism for regulation of the β_2AR or other G protein-coupled receptors. In certain cell types, receptor gene transcription is probably affected.

iii) Gene transcription: Down-regulated induced by prolonged receptor stimulation can reduce transcription rates of receptor gene [11, 13]. In some cases, such as for the β_2AR, short term agonist stimulation increases the rate of gene transcription [10]. It is known that the transcriptional regulation of a variety of genes is mediated through a CRE present in their promotor region [14], recognized by CREB, a transcription factor whose ability to stimulate target gene transcription is regulated by phosphorylation [14, 15]. Using β_2AR promoter-CAT reporter gene construct and site-directed mutagenesis experiments, we have shown that the β_2AR gene expression is sensitive to the activity of CREB transcription factor system [10]. This CRE sequence binds the CREB transcription factor, and mutation of this sequence abolishes cAMP stimulation of expression and dramatically reduces basal level expression from the promoter [16]. An additional level of complexity in the manner by which cAMP dependent genes are regulated is indicated by the discovery of CREM (cAMP-responsive element modulator), a gene with sequence similarities to CREB. Splice variants of the CREM gene can generate protein products capable of binding CREs in either a stimulatory or inhibitory fashion [6, 17]. This raises the possibility that up- and downregulation of β_2AR gene transcription could proceed through the same sequence element. We are attempting to explore this possibility.

Short- vs. long-acting β-agonists

The term of "short" and "long" is used to indicate the duration of the β-agonists as evaluated by the responsiveness of effector, in this case, the activity of adenylyl cyclase, following receptor activation. A short-acting β-agonist may be capable of causing both uncoupling and down-regulation in vitro, depending upon the length of time of exposure. However, in vivo, there is little evidence of significant desensitization. By contrast, the major concern for long-acting β-agonists is the potential for substantial desensitization, due to a relatively long residence time at the receptor. Indeed, prolonged exposure to β-agonists in vivo has been shown to lead to β_2AR down-regulation in the airway [18–20]. Great effort has been made to circumvent this problem by searching for β-agonists that provide prolonged coverage (e.g. hours of targeted functional activity) in the treatment of asthma without producing tachyphylaxis. One of the well-known long-acting β-agonists recently developed is salmeterol, a selective β_2-agonist. This compound has the unique ability to remain efficacious over many hours as a long-acting relaxant of airway smooth muscle for asthma therapy without apparently causing desensitization [21–23]. However, the molecular mechanism underlying the long-duration property of salmeterol is unclear. Since the human bronchial epithelial cell line BEAS-2B has been widely used as an in vitro model for understanding regulation of the β_2AR in the human airway, this cell line was chosen to directly examine the effect of the long-acting β_2-agonist salmeterol, in comparison with the non-selective and shorter-acting β-agonist isoprotenerol, on β_2AR expression and function.

Experimental findings

Since appears that lower concentrations of salmeterol are more therapeutically relevant, we used 10 nM of salmeterol and isoprotenerol on the following experiments. Treatment of BEAS-2B cells with isoprotenerol induced a rapid and transient increase of adenylyl cyclase activity that is the typical pattern to continuous β-agonist exposure [7]. The cAMP produced was maximized around 30 minutes and declined rapidly by 8 hours [24]. Salmeterol showed a similar pattern of response as isoprotenerol. However, the overall amount of cAMP generated by salmeterol was lower. This is likely due to the fact that salmeterol is a partial agonist, as compared with isoprotenerol, which is a full agonist [24–27]. Similar to previous reports, β_2AR desensitization occurs in BEAS-2B cells in response to isoprotenerol [28, 29], even at a concentration of 10 nM [24]. This was conclusion was based upon an examination of

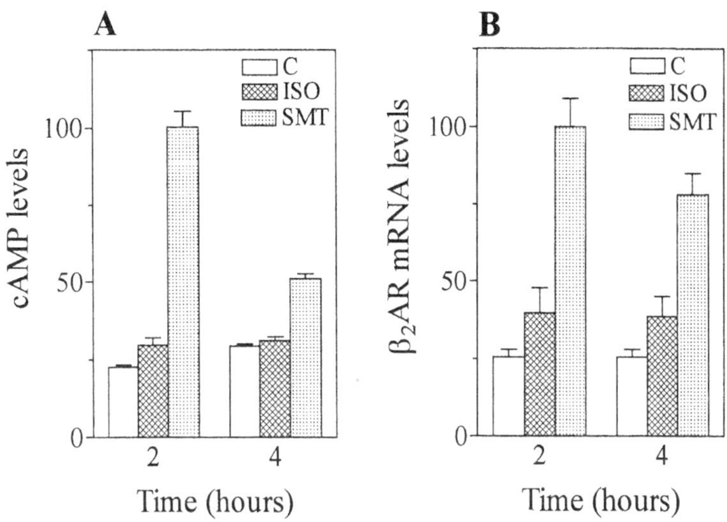

Fig. 3. The long-acting properties of salmeterol, in comparison to isoprotenerol, in response to a brief exposure to the β-agonists (10 nM) in human bronchial epithelial cell line BEAS-2B cells. Ten minutes after the treatment, the medium containing the agonist was removed. The cells were washed and replaced with fresh medium without agonist. The cellular levels of cAMP (***A***) and β_2AR mRNA (***B***) were measured after the wash at the times indicated. It clearly demonstrated that the adenylyl cyclase activity and β_2AR gene expression are higher in the salmeterol- than in the isoprotenerol-treated cells. *C* control; *ISO* isoprotenerol; *SMT* salmeterol

both β_2AR gene expression by RNase prodection, and by measuring adenylyl cyclase activity. However, treatment of BEAS-2B cells with 10 nM salmeterol had no such down-regulator effect [24].

To explore further the long-acting characteristics of salmeterol, the experiments employed a 10 minute transient exposure regimen which may reflect the in vivo situation more closely. It clearly demonstrates that salmeterol, but not isoprotenerol, is able to persistently elevate both intracellular cAMP production and β_2AR mRNA transcripts, even as along as four hours after the agonist has been removed from the medium (Fig. 3). This persistent elevation of steady-state levels of β_2AR mRNA most likely results from the increased cAMP-dependent synthesis of new transcripts via the CREB transcription factor system [16].

Regardless of the mechanism involved, these data suggest that the long-acting characteristics of salmeterol are, at least in part, due to the ability of this agonist to maintain a population of functional β_2AR through persistent elevation of β_2AR gene transcription. This molecular information of salmeterol could make a better understanding of the long-lasting β-agonist that may enhance the design of much longer-duration of β_2-agonist for the treatment of asthma.

References

1. Dixon RAF, Kobilka BK et al (1986) Cloning of the gene and cDNA for mammalian β-adrenergic receptor and homology with rhodopsin. Nature 321: 75–79
2. Dohlman HG, Thorner J, Caron MG, Lefkowitz RJ (1991) Model systems for the study of seven-transmembrane-segment receptors. Annu Rev Biochem 60: 653–688
3. Pitcher JA, Inglese J, Higgins JB et al (1992) Role of βγ subunits of G proteins in targeting the β-adrenergic receptor kinase to membrane-bound receptors. Science 257: 1267–1274
4. Simonds WF, Maji HK, Garrison A (1993) G proteins and βARK: a new twist for the coiled coil. Trends Biochem Sci 18: 317
5. Lefkowitz RJ, Hausdorff WP, Caron MG (1990) Role of phosphorylation in desensitization of the β-adrenoceptor. Trends Pharmacol Sci 11: 190–194
6. Collins S, Caron MG, Lefkowitz RJ (1991) Regulation of adrenergic receptor responsiveness through modulation of receptor gene expression. Annu Rev Physiol 53: 497–508
7. Hausdorff WP, Caron MG, Lefkowitz RJ (1990) Turning off the signal: desensitization of β-adrenergic receptor function. FASEB J 4: 2881–2889
8. Inglese J, Glickman JF, Lorenz W, Caron MG, Lefkowitz RJ (1992) Isoprenylation of a protein kinase: requirement of farnesylation/α-carboxyl methylation for full enzymatic activity of rhodopsin kinase. J Biol Chem 267: 1422–1425
9. Hadcock JR, Wang H, Malbon CC (1989) Agonist-induced destabilization of beta-adrenergic receptor mRNA. Attenuation of glucocorticoid induced up-regulation of β-adrenergic receptors. J Biol Chem 264: 19928–19933
10. Collins S, Bouvier M, Bolanowsky MA, Caron MG, Lefkowitz RJ (1989) Cyclic AMP stimulates transcription of the β_2-adrenergic receptor gene in response to short term agonist exposure. Proc Natl Acad Sci USA 86: 4853–4857
11. Saji M, Akamizu T, Sanchez M, Obici S, Avvedimento E, Gottesman ME,

Kohn LD (1992) Regulation of thyrotropin receptor gene expression in rat FRTL-5 thyroid cells. Endocrinol 130: 520–533
12. Ihara H, Nakanishi S (1990) Selective inhibition of expression of the substance P receptor mRNA in pancreatic acinar AR42J cells by glucocorticoids. J Biol Chem 265: 22441–22445
13. Habecker BA, Nathanson NM (1992) Regulation of muscarinic acetylcholine receptor mRNA expression by activation of homologous and heterologous receptors. Proc Natl Acad Sci USA 89: 5035–5038
14. Montiminy MR, Gonzalez GA, Yamamoto KK (1990) Regulation of cAMP-inducible genes by CREB. Trends Neurosci 13: 184–188
15. Hoeffler JP, Habener JF (1990) Characterization of a cyclic AMP regulatory element DNA-binding protein. Trends Endocrinol Metab Jan/Feb, 155–158
16. Collins S, Altshmied J, Herbsman O, Caron MG, Mellon PL, Lefkowitz RJ (1990) A cAMP response element in the β_2-adrenergic receptor gene confers transcriptional autoregulation by cAMP. J Biol Chem 265: 19330–19335
17. Foulkes NS, Sassone-Corsi P (1992) More is better: activators and repressors from the same gene. Cell 68: 411–414
18. Nishikawa M, Mark JC, Shirasaki H, Barnes PJ (1993) Differential downregulation of pulmonary β_1- and β_2-adrenoceptor messenger RNA with prolonged in vivo infusion of isoprenaline. Eur J Pharmacol 247: 131–138
19. Nishikawa M, Mark JC, Shirasaki H, Barnes PJ (1994) Long-term exposure to norepinephrine results in down-regulation and reduced mRNA expression of pulmonary beta-adrenergic receptors in guinea pigs. Am J Respir Cell Mol Biol 10: 91–99
20. Turki J, Green SA, Newman KB, Meyers MA, Liggett SB (1995) Human lung cell β_2-adrenergic receptors desensitize in response to in vivo administered β-agonist. Am J Physiol 269: L709–L714
21. Johnson M, Butchers PR, Coleman RA, Nials AT et al (1993) The pharmacology of salmeterol. Life Sci 52: 2131–2143
22. Johnson M (1995) Pharmacology of long-acting β-agonists. Ann Allergy Asthma Immunol 75: 177–179
23. Anderson GP, Linden A, Rabe KF (1994) Why are long-acting beta-adrenoceptor agonist long-acting? Eur Respir J 7: 569–578
24. Wang S, Johnson M, Collins S (1997) Persistent up-regulation of the β_2AR-adenylyl cyclase system by the long-acting β-agonist salmeterol (in preparation)
25. McCrea KE, Hill SJ (1993) Salmeterol, a long-acting β_2-adrenoceptor agonist mediating cyclic AMP accumulation in a neuronal cell line. Br J Pharmacol 110: 619–626
26. Clark RB, Allal C, Friedman J, Johnson M, Barber R (1996) Stable activation and desensitization of β_2-adrenergic receptor stimulation of adenylyl

cyclase by salmeterol: evidence for Quasi-irreversible binding to an exosite. Mol Pharmacol 49: 182–189
27. McCrea KE, Hill SJ (1996) Comparison of duration of agonist action at β_1- and β_2-adrenoceptors in C6 glioma cells: evidence that long duration of action of salmeterol is specific to the β_2-adrenoceptor. Mol Pharmacol 49: 927–937
28. Penn RB, Kelson SG, Benovic JL (1994) Regulation of β-agonist- and prostaglandin E_2-mediated adenylyl cyclase activity in human airway epithelial cells. Am J Respir Cell Mol Biol 11: 496–505
29. Mardini IA, Higgins NC, Zhou S, Benovic JL, Kelsen SG (1994) Functional behaviour of the β-adrenergic receptor-adenylyl cyclase system in rabbit airway epithelium. Am J Respir Cell Mol Biol 11: 287–295

Correspondence: Dr. Sheila Collins, Duke University Medical Center, Division of Biological Psychiatry and Pharmacology, S.W. Stedman Center for Nutritional Studies, Box 3557, Durham, North Carolina 27710, U.S.A.

Discussion

Dr. Block: I would like to ask three questions, if you don't mind. One relates to the last point. You mentioned that PDE is essentially involved to some degree in the ability of salmeterol to prolong the activity of the beta-2-adrenergic receptors. As we all know, there are various isoforms of the PDE and it could well be that salmeterol, depending on its CAMP-specific activity, is capable of affecting one of those.

Dr. Collins: Well, we haven't looked for exactly which forms of the PDE's are expressed, for example in the B-2-B cells. Two of the forms, I recall, can be very dramatically stimulated in their expression by cyclic AMP, but naturally this would then depress the level of cyclic AMP further over a prolonged period of time. I think it would be interesting for us to go back and see in all of our samples which PDE and whether those levels change at all. I think that any effect of salmeterol, though, would be primarily at the level of the receptor itself. And so then, the ability of the cell to produce and maintain a certain level of cyclic AMP is certainly going to be a balance between whatever PDE's are there and the degree of agonist activation of the pathway.

Dr. Block: In addition you mentioned PKA analogous to PKC. Is there evidence that certain isoforms exist, because it could also well be that one of those isoforms may be affected by salmeterol and related adrenergic agonists.

Dr. Collins: Right. There is some evidence that the receptor, at least in an in vitro situation could be phosphorylated by PKC, but you know, almost anything in a test tube can be phosphorylated by PKC. We have not looked as to which forms are there. It would certainly be quite easy to do, since my husband has prepared anti-sera to every single PKC that exists, so we could very easily examine it, but we just have not, yet. We've really just focused on this small defined area.

Dr. Block: Coming to molecular biology, by using antisense oligonucleotides against CREB, could you completely block reactivation of the gene-encoding beta-adrenergic?

Dr. Collins: Right. I think the first thing to do, though, would be to see which forms are there, because now the CREB family has become quite large. Thanks to the work done by Paolo Sassoni-Corsi in Strasbourg, they bear some tremendous homology, so you first would need to know what you were dealing with and then, if you may be able to specifically block one or the other. Since antisense methods are still a bit empirical, I somewhat favour the approach of transfecting genes into the cells to examine the potential roles that way, and that's the approach that we're currently taking in the lab, but we don't have specific answers to that yet.

Dr. Gary Anderson (Basel): A question about the copy number of beta-2 receptors in relation to auto-regulation mechanisms: Epithelial cells express many beta-2 receptors, whereas airway smooth muscle seems to express far fewer beta-2 receptors per cell.

Dr. Collins: Well, in the B-2-B cells, the level of expression of the beta-2 receptors is really rather low. It's probably between 50 and 90 fmol/mg receptor protein, which is not a lot. I don't know how this relates to the numbers of beta-2 receptors on human airway smooth muscle. Maybe someone can tell me the answer to that. But you know, I think the fact that we're looking at a level of receptor that is so low makes this model quite relevant. It was actually a significant problem in doing some of the experiments because we'd need so many cells to simply do, for example, one immunoprecipitation. So I think we're looking at a reasonable situation.

Dr. Pohl (Vienna): Have you looked at other cells, especially human epithelial cells of normals and asthmatics? Do you think that there is a difference in the activation of the beta-2 receptor gene?

Dr. Collins: I wouldn't be surprised, since, when we first reported that there were changes in beta-2 receptor expression by cyclic AMP, later there were reports that some of the down-regulation of the receptor appears to involve a change in receptor message half-life, but also in a hamster smooth muscle line, in other cells when you look, for example, in A431 cells, you can find no evidence of change in receptor message half-life but a complete repression of transcription. So I think from cell to cell, (and there is also evidence from Dr. Barnes' group), that different types of cells expressing the beta-2 regulate that receptor or transcribe that gene in slightly different ways. Sometimes you read a paper and a person tells you, okay you know, this is how the experiment was and therefore this is how it must be in every cell. I think that's a dangerous conclusion to draw.

Dr. W. Pohl: I know. But in particular I am asking about human epithelial cells gained by brushings, by bronchoscopy. Do you breed them and then look for the gene expression?

Dr. Collins: We haven't done this kind of experiment. I mean our goal has been to just try to understand, with these kinds of molecular tools, what is reasonably possible in a reasonably good model cell line. I hope someone will do your experiment, however.

Molecular interactions between glucocorticoids and β_2-agonists

I. M. Adcock and *D. A. Stevens*

Department of Thoracic Medicine, Imperial College School of Medicine at NHLI, London, U. K.

Summary

Glucocorticoids and β_2-agonists may regulate gene transcription in a cell- and gene-specific manner at both the transcriptional and post-transcriptional level. For this transcription factor interaction to be of importance in asthma, it must occur in a cell or cells which are key targets for steroids and which also express surface β_2-receptors and respond to β_2-agonist stimulation with elevation of cAMP. Many pulmonary cells express β_2-receptors and these same cells express GR. Airway epithelial cells, T-lymphocytes and macrophages are target cells an which this effect may be of therapeutic relevance, particularly as all produce cytokines which may orchestrate or perpetuate the allergic inflammatory response.

Asthma is due to a chronic inflammation of the airways and glucocorticoids are the most effective therapy currently available for the control of asthmatic inflammation. Indeed, inhaled steroids have now become the mainstay of chronic asthma therapy. Whereas β-agonists are most effective in treating the airways constriction associated with the onset of asthma symptoms and are often the only drug prescribed for the treatment of mild asthmatics although even at this stage of the disease there may well be ongoing, possibly irreversible, inflammatory changes in the airway [1]. β-Adrenoreceptor agonists and glucocorticoids are the two most effective treatments for asthma and are often used in combination. In this chapter we summarise the interactions between these drugs at a biochemical and molecular level and discuss the possible consequences for asthma therapy.

Mechanisms of glucocorticoid action

Glucocorticoids have been proposed to mediate their anti-inflammatory responses, not against the source of the stress itself, but by preventing the body's normal reactions to stress, preventing those reactions from overshooting and threatening homeostasis [2]. Thus, many of the physiological and pharmacological effects of glucocorticoids may be secondary to modulation of the action of numerous inter- and intracellular mediators including other hormones, prostaglandins, lymphokines and bioactive peptides. Glucocorticoids act by influencing transcription of target genes [3]. Glucocorticoids freely diffuse into the cell from the surrounding milieu and bind to the 94 kDa glucocorticoid receptor (GR), which is held in an inactive form within the cytoplasm by the presence of 2 molecules of the molecular chaperone hsp90. Upon ligand binding the GR undergoes a conformational change resulting in dissociation of the hsp90 proteins and unmasking of a nuclear localisation signal. The steroid-GR complex translocates into the nucleus where it may bind directly to glucocorticoid responsive elements (GREs) on DNA in the promoter region of steroid sensitive genes. Alternatively, the steroid-receptor complex may form heterologous complexes with other DNA-binding proteins, so modulating an effect that they would otherwise have on gene transcription [4]. An interaction between the pro-inflammatory transcription factors activating protein-1 (AP-1) and nuclear factor kappa B (NF-κB) and GR has been demonstrated in cultured cells [5, 6], in human peripheral blood cells [7] and in human lung [8, 9] and may be an important aspect of the anti-inflammatory effect of steroids [10] (Fig. 1). Recent data suggests that transactivation by nuclear hormone receptors such as GR depends upon the co-activator CREB-binding protein (CBP), or the related P300 protein, to trigger

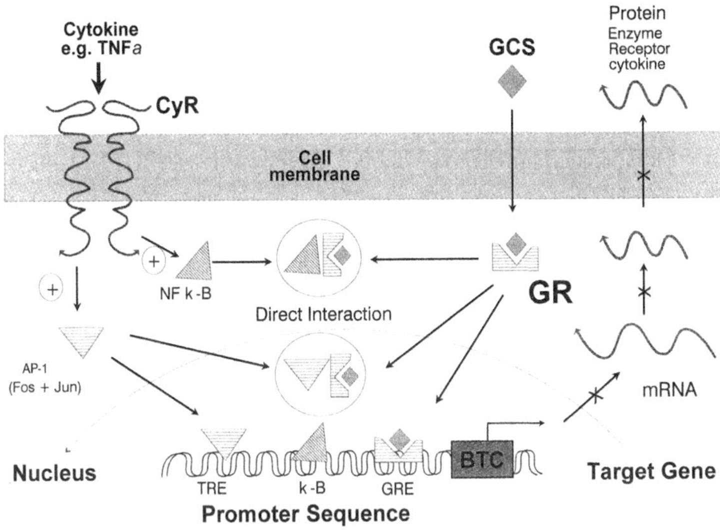

Fig. 1. The mechanism of glucocorticoid action. Glucocorticosteroids *(GCS)* freely diffuse from the circulation across cell membranes where they interact with a glucocorticoid receptor *(GR)*. Upon ligand binding the receptor is activated and translocated to the nucleus where it can bind to specific DNA sequences *(GRE)* upstream of the start site of transcription. This causes bending of the DNA and interaction of the DNA-bound GR with the basal transcription complex *(BTC)* and modulation of target gene transcription. Alternatively GCS may act by inhibiting the ability of other transcription factors to bind to DNA. AP-1 and NF-κB activated by cytokines or other inflammatory mediators via specific receptors (e. g. cytokine receptors, CyR) may interact with activated GR and either prevent DNA binding directly or interfere with AP-1 or NF-κB interaction with the BTC causing inhibition of inflammatory gene transcription

RNA polymerase II and hence modulate gene transcription [11–15]. CBP and P300 are very large having the ability to interact with a variety of different transcription factors and also with components of the basal transcriptional machinery. These steroid receptors/CBP/P300 interactions are greatly enhanced by ligand binding. The steroid receptor/CBP/P300 complex may also interact with a variety of other activating or silencing mediators thus forming a ternary complex bound to DNA. Thus multiple co-activators may jointly modulate transactivation mediated by a single DNA binding transcription factor. The

GR/AP-1 and GR/NF-κB interactions may both be mediated via CBP/P300 as the common intermediary molecule.

In asthma glucocorticoids exert effects on expression of a wide variety of genes, including those for cytokines, receptors and enzymes, all of which are regulated by a variety of second messenger signals, but the absolute and relative importance of any of these mediators to the therapeutic response is not yet clear.

Mechanisms of β-agonist action

β-Adrenoceptors (βR) in human airway smooth muscle are of the β_2-receptor subtype [16] and so selective β_2-agonists are used to counteract airway constriction in asthmatic patients. Following ligand binding to the receptor, receptor-associated G_S proteins are activated and couple with adenylyl cyclase (AC) [17]. The coupling of activated G_S and AC leads to enhanced production of cAMP and subsequent activation of cAMP-dependent protein kinase A (PKA). PKA then phosphorylates and thus inactivates myosin light chain kinase (MLCK) preventing myosin phosphorylation. Concomitant activation of Ca^{2+}-Mg^{2+}-ATPases in the endoplasmic reticulum and plasma membrane [18] decreases Ca^{2+} levels thereby reducing Ca^{2+}-dependent actin-myosin interactions and leading to relaxation of airway smooth muscle. It has also been proposed that β-agonists may also cause airway smooth muscle relaxation through a cAMP-independent mechanism via direct coupling between the receptor-activated G_S (α_S) protein and a large conductance Ca^{2+}-activated potassium channel leading to cell hyperpolarization and hence smooth muscle relaxation [19]. Thus low doses of β-adrenoceptor agonists may cause airway bronchodilation without elevation of intracellular cAMP.

β-adrenoceptor agonists may also influence gene transcription through elevation of cyclic 3′,5′ adenosine monophosphate (cAMP) and activation of PKA [20]. cAMP mediates the hormonal stimulation of a variety of eukaryotic genes through a conserved cAMP response element (CRE) [21]. Transcriptional induction by cAMP is rapid, peaking at 30 minutes and declining gradually over 24 hours [22]. This burst in transcription is resistant to inhibitors of protein synthesis,

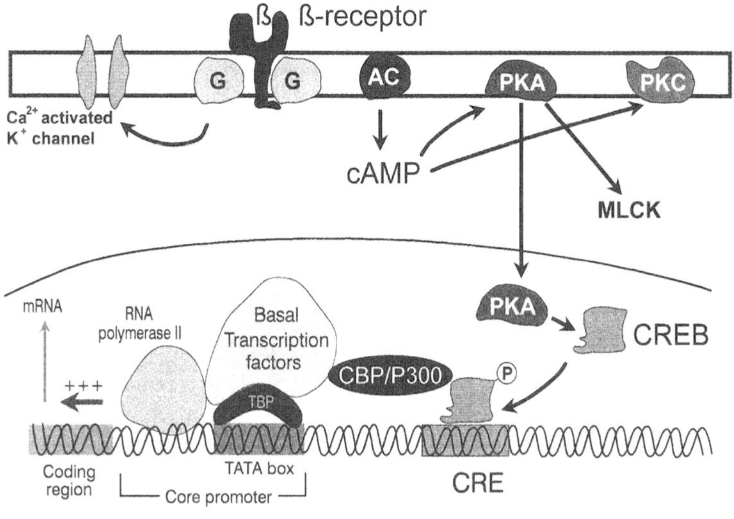

Fig. 2. The mechanism of β_2-agonist action. Ligand binding to the β_2-receptor causes airway smooth muscle relaxation. This may occur through a variety of mechanisms. Induction of cAMP following activation of cAMP-dependent protein kinase A *(PKA)* may lead to phosphorylation of a number of proteins including myosin light chain kinase *(MLCK),* alteration in Ca^{++} levels and subsequent inhibition of smooth muscle contraction. Alternatively direct coupling between the receptor-activated G_s (α_s) protein *(G)* and a large conductance Ca^{2+}-activated potassium channel may lead to cell hyperpolarization and smooth muscle relaxation.

β_2-Agonists may also affect gene transcription. Activation of receptor-associated G_s proteins and coupling with adenylyl cyclase *(AC)* leads to enhanced production of cAMP and subsequent activation of PKA. Activation of PKA leads to translocation of the C-subunit to the nucleus and subsequent phosphorylation of the cAMP response element binding protein *(CREB)* enhancing its interaction with specific DNA binding sites (CRE). CREB interacts with the BTM through its associtated binding protein CBP, or other signal transducing proteins such as P300. These proteins allow signals to be passed to the basal transcription factors sitting above the TATA promoter signal on DNA (TATA box) linked via the TATA box binding protein *(TBP).* Regulation of which modulates mRNA production through the action of RNA polymerase II

suggesting that cAMP may stimulate gene expression by inducing the covalent modification rather than de novo synthesis of specific nuclear factors. Treatment of cells with cAMP causes translocation of the catalytic subunit (C-subunit) of PKA to the nucleus [23] where it phosphorylates serine-133 on the cAMP response element binding protein (CREB) enhancing its DNA-binding and transactivating activity [21]. CREB mediates its transactivating abilities via an associated binding protein (CBP) which transduces the CREB signal to the transcription initiation complex [24]. Activated CREB may persist for prolonged periods within the nucleus and therefore even a brief exposure to β-adrenoceptor agonist may lead to a prolonged effect on transcription. cAMP may also interfere with the effects of PKC activation through inhibition of mitogen activated protein kinase (MAPK) [25–28] (Fig. 2).

The precise mode of CREB action in modulation gene transcription is made more complex by the existence of a large number of CREB isoforms all capable of forming distinct hetero- and homo-dimers with other isoforms and with other bZIP proteins such as AP-1 [26, 29]. Also included within the CREB family of transcription factors are the group of modulators (CREMs) which repress gene activation by CREB and which bind at the same CRE sites [30].

The rate of transcription of the β_2R gene is increased in response to β-adrenergic agonist stimulation of the receptor at the cell surface. This positive autoregulation of the β_2-adrenergic receptor gene appears to occur through receptor-mediated stimulation of adenylyl cyclase, with consequent activation of CREB and stimulation of β_2-adrenergic receptor gene transcription [31, 32]. However, most long term exposure to β-agonists results in decreased mRNA in cell lines and in lung in vivo [33–35]. This reduced expression of β_2-receptors is due to reduced gene transcription and is associated with a reduction in CREB activity and may be related to receptor desensitization or internalisation [35].

Effect of glucocorticoids on β_2-receptors

a) Upregulation of receptor number

Dexamethasone, a synthetic glucocorticoid, increases the number of β_2-R in human lung measured by radioligand binding [36]. Several putative GREs have been identified in the promoter sequence of the human β_2-R gene [37] and increased β_2R gene transcription occurs following dexamethasone treatment through a GRE in the 5′-flanking region of the gene [38] in human lung tissue. This occurred in both a time and dose-dependent manner which was consistent with the later induction of receptor binding activity [34] (Fig. 3). This confirmed earlier reports of a similar action of dexamcthasone on β_2R in cultured cell lines [33]. The mRNA half-life and stability is tissue- and cell-specific and is determined to some extent by the level of RNase activity in the cytoplasm of each particular cell type. However, dexamethasone has not been found to alter the half-life of β_2R message [34]. The efficiency of coupling between the β_2R and G_s (the G protein that mediates stimulation of AC has been reported to be modulated by glucocorticoids [39]. As a result, β_2R-stimulated AC activity and cAMP accumulation increase following glucocorticoid treatment. Animals that have been depleted of glucocorticoids by adrenalectomy, in contrast, lose their ability to maintain the sensitivity of the βR-coupled AC cyclase system [33].

b) Inhibition of down-regulation

Chronic administration of β_2-agonists in animals *in vivo* causes a marked down-regulation of β_2-R as measured by mRNA and ligand

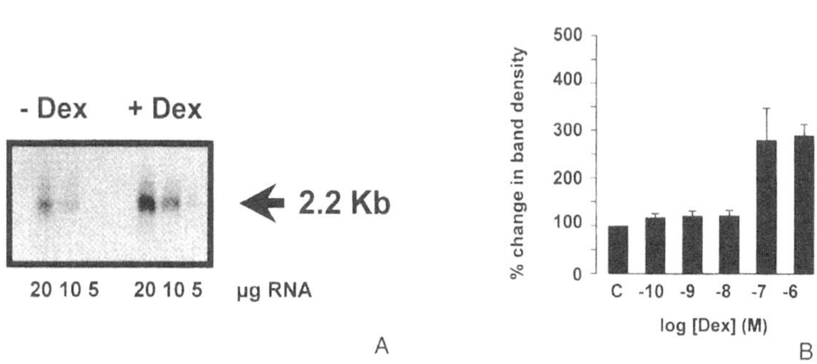

Fig. 3. Effect of glucocorticoids on β_2-receptor expression. Dexamethasone induced an upregulation of β_2-receptor mRNA as measured by Northern blot analysis (left hand panel) and expression of the β_2-receptor as measured by Western blot analysis (right hand panel). This increase in β_2-receptor expression occurs through a direct action of the activated glucocorticoid receptor on positive GREs within the promoter region of the β_2-receptor gene

binding in human [34] and rat [40] lung in a cell specific manner with less effect in airway smooth muscle than in lung parenchyma [35]. This agonist promoted down-regulation of β_2R may be reversed by treatment with glucocorticoids [36]. Thus in human lung, neutrophils and lymphocytes glucocorticoids induce an increase in the synthesis of β_2-R [36]. Autoradiographic mapping studies in rat indicate that glucocorticoids up regulate β_2-receptors and prevent down-regulation of β_2-receptors in all cell types, including airway smooth muscle cells [40]. Such an effect may have clinical implications for preventing the development of tolerance to β_2-agonists in asthmatic patients treated with β-agonists.

Chronic β-agonist therapy in asthmatic subjects results in reduction in βR density in circulating polymorphonuclear leukocytes and lymphocytes [41] and the down-regulated β_2R number is restored with oral prednisone. However, a difference in susceptibility to down-regulation between lung and lymphoid tissue has been reported [42].

Interactions of GR with other transcription factors

Recent studies have provided increasing evidence for functional interactions between the family of nuclear hormone receptors, which includes the steroid, vitamin D and thyroid hormone receptors, and other transcription factors not involving a natural promoter [3]. This is particularly the case with glucocorticoid-inducible genes, which frequently show GREs contiguous with DNA regulatory sequences for other transcription factors in the promoter region. These include binding sites for SP1, NF1, CACCC and CCAAT box binding proteins [43, 44], CREB [45–47] and AP-I factors [5, 9], or a second GRE [43, 44]. The effect of these other factors can lead to either enhancement or repression of gene transcription driven by the glucocorticoids. GR has been shown to repress gene expression by functional interference with several different transcriptional activators [5–7, 45–47]. For instance, repression of osteocalcin, proliferin and collagenase gene expression by glucocorticoids is due to inhibition at an AP-I site by a different mechanism involving a protein-protein interaction between the subunits of AP-1 and GR mediated through the transcriptional accessory protein CBP leading to a mutual inhibition of their transcriptional and DNA binding activities [11–15, 48, 49].

NF-κB, an important mediator of many inflammatory genes, is also supressed by glucocorticoids in a manner analogous to that shown for AP-1 with a direct protein-protein interaction being shown between GR and the p65 subunit of the dimeric NF-κB molecule. Examples of this have been demonstrated for the regulation of several genes including those for IL-6 [6], IL-8 [50] and COX-2 [51]. The major mechanism of GR action being the ability to disrupt NF-κB interaction with or signal transduction to the transcription initiation complex possibly via mutual competition for CBP rather than DNA binding per se.

In some instances CBP can be a limiting component in the cell allowing cross talk between different signalling pathways such as that between nuclear receptors and AP-1. AP-1 activity is inhibited by nuclear receptors, such as GR and retinoic acid receptors and over-expression of CBP or P300 overcomes this inhibition [12].

Conversely the function of nuclear hormone receptors can also be impaired by sequestration of CBP/P300. Phosphorylation of CREB by PKA enables CREB to interact with CBP and hence interfere with retinoic acid- and thyroid hormone-induced gene transcription. Furthermore, different nuclear hormone receptors can antagonise one another in a ligand-dependent manner. Thus competition for limiting co-factors, such as CBP or P300, may contribute to the control of gene transcription (Fig. 4).

Protein kinase activators such as cAMP can induce transcription mediated by nuclear receptors, either autonomously or synergistically with hormone (PR and ER). This may occur by direct phosphorylation of the receptor or by phosphorylation of the co-activator CBP by MAPK or PKA which has been shown to enhance the co-activation potential of CBP. Interestingly both oestrogen and progesterone can induce the phosphorylation of CREB possibly by increasing cAMP levels. Phosphorylated CREB could then sequester CBP/P300 and negatively interfere with the action of the steroid hormone receptors. This may be balanced by the enhancement of CBP interaction upon hormone binding and also by the phosphorylation of the steroid receptor and/or CBP by PKA. Thus the signalling pathways are interconnected

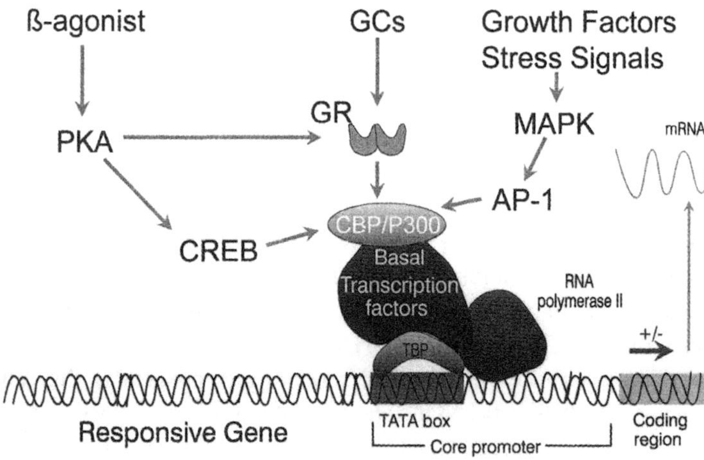

Fig. 4. Mechanism of potential interactions of the glucocorticoid receptor *(GR)* with β-agonist-induced transcription factor *(CREB)* and transducing proteins (CBP and P300). CREB modulation of gene transcription occurs following CREB phosphorylation and activation by protein kinase A *(PKA)* and subsequent interaction with CBP (or P300) leading to induction of RNA polymerase II activity following modulation of the basal transcription factors. The basal transcription factors are bought together at the start site of transcription by binding of TATA binding protein *(TBP)* to a specific sequence in the promoter DNA known as the TATA box. The activated glucocorticoid adtivity *(GR)* also regulates gene transcription via DNA binding and subsequent modulation of RNA polymerase activity through association with CBP or P300. Thus competition for the co-activator may cause mutual inhibition of β-agonist and glucocorticoid activities. This effect may be modulated by PKA phosphorylation of GR increasing GR transactivating potential or by other molecules interacting with the large CBP of P300 molecules. These include AP-1 activated by cytokines, growth factors and stress signals or other activators of mitogen activated protein kinase (MAPK) cascades

in an intricate network involving the promiscuous co-activators CBP and P300 whose ability to form multi-protein complexes are an essential factor in integrating many signal pathways.

Actions of cAMP elevating agents on steroid actions

As shown above there is a great potential for interactions between GR and either β_2-agonists or drugs that increase cAMP of CREB levels. The exact functional response elicited by specific cells in response to these stimuli will therefore depend upon the relative importance and levels of expression of the multiple components of these signal pathways and their associated transcription factors or accessory proteins. Here we will give examples of functional and biochemical readouts of these interactions, hopefully, showing that these effects are both cell and context specific and also depend on the dose of β_2-agonist/cAMP elevating agent used.

Synergy

Synergy between the GR and other transcription factors was first reported for NFI, SPI and CACCC binding proteins in genes encoding tyrosine aminotransferase and rat tryptophan oxygenase. Functional co-operativity in these instances was shown to be critically dependent on the spacing between the regulatory elements but not their orientation and is mediated by protein-protein interaction rather than co-coperative DNA binding [43, 44]. This suggests a basic model of glucocorticoid-induced transcriptional activation requiring multiple GREs or a combination of a GRE with other transcription factor-binding sites for constitution of a hormone-inducible enhancer.

Both dexamethasone and forskolin, a direct activator of AC, modulate neurotensin (NT) production from rat hypothalamic neurones in primary culture. Dexamethasone gave a dose-dependent increase in NT content with a maximum at 1μM whilst forskolin (1μM) alone had no effect on either the content or the number of immunoreactive NT cells. However, co-treatment with dexamethasone and forskolin, both at 1 μM, caused a 3-fold increase in NT content and a 4-fold increase in cell number when compared to dexamethasone alone. This synergistic increase was mediated at the transcriptional level [52].

Dexamethasone (0.1 μM) transiently increases tissue-type plasminogen activator (tPA) mRNA accumulation 2-fold in rat hepatoma cells, whereas incubation with the cAMP analogue, 8-Br-cAMP (1 mM), alone results in a sustained 2-fold increase. Combined 8Br-cAMP and dexamethasone treatment causes a 10–15-fold increase in mRNA levels. This induction of tPA gene transcription requires concomitant protein synthesis and occurs, at least in part at the transcriptional level. Furthermore, the action of dexamethasone must precede that of 8Br-cAMP and requires ongoing protein synthesis, whereas the action of 8Br-cAMP has no such requirement [53].

Incubation of rabbit amnion cells with cortisol (20 nM) for 24 hours induces a 16–18-fold increase in oxytocin receptors (OTR) in vitro. The effects of cortisol were dose- and steroid-dependent. Addition of 50 μM forskolin to the dexamethasone in the cell culture medium induced a large, up to 182-fold, increase in OTR expression. These effects were inhibited by activation of PKC [54].

Addition

Lymphocyte activation, proliferation and some effector functions are regulated by glucocorticoids and elevations of intracellular cyclic AMP. Treatment of resting human lymphocytes with dexamethasone (0.1 μM), sensitised prostaglandin E_2 stimulated cyclic AMP accumulation in a time- and concentration-dependent manner and enhanced inhibition of concanavalin A-induced Ca^{2+} elevation. In contrast, β_2-adrenoceptor density, immunodetectable α-subunits of the G-proteins, Gs and Gi, and pertussis toxin substrates were not significantly altered by dexamethasone treatment. From these studies it was demonstrated that dexamethasone treatment sensitises cyclic AMP formation in resting human lymphocytes by altering AC rather than G-proteins or hormone receptors. This results in an enhanced capability of cyclic AMP generating agonists to inhibit early steps of lymphocyte activation [55].

The somatostatin gene (SS) is transcriptional regulated via a CRE element. cAMP and forskolin stimulated SS gene transcription 4–5 fold in PC12 cells whilst dexamethasone (1 μM) alone produced a dose-dependent 2-fold stimulation of SS gene transcription. Dexamethasone (1 μM) exerted an additive effect on 1.5 mM cAMP-induced SS gene transcription which was dependent on PKA activity. An effect which was mimicked by 10 μM foskolin. The stimulatory effects of dexamethasone were removed upon deletion of the promoter fragment 250 to –71 (a region that does not contain a GRE) but did not affect cAMP action. These studies showed that glucocorticoid-induced transactivation was mediated via protein-protein interactions between GR and CREB and CREB-related binding proteins [56].

Glucocorticoids induce a down-regulation of GR in rat HTC cells. Forskolin (25 μM) and 8Br-cAMP (50 μM) prevents this action by increasing the levels of both [^{3}H]dexamethasone binding capacity and GR mRNA by increasing GR mRNA half-life and phosphorylation state [57]. This results in enhancement of GR transcriptional activation.

In a human breast carcinoma-derived cell line, T47D(A1–2), containing a hormone-responsive luciferase reporter gene, manipulation of cell growth conditions or cellular signal transduction in a variety of ways can enhance or impair glucocorticoid-mediated induction of a target gene [58]. The 4-fold induction by dexamethasone (0.1 μM) could be further enhanced 2- to 3-fold by co-addition of 8Br-cAMP (1 mM). Treatment with 1 μM forskolin, a direct activator of adenylate cyclase, also enhanced the hormone-induced level of luciferase approximately 2-fold in a dose-dependent manner. Forskolin had no effect in the absence of hormone. In contrast, activating PKA by inhibiting cAMP turnover with the phosphodiesterase inhibitors isobutylmethylxanthine (IBMX) or Ro20-1724, both at 500 μM, inhibited the hormone response rather than potentiated it.

A direct interaction between GR and CREB, whilst bound to DNA regulates the expression of the PEPCK gene, which encodes the rate-limiting enzyme in gluceogenesis [59]. 0.1 mM cAMP induced a 5-fold induction of PEPCK mRNA in H4IIE rat hepatoma cells which was similar to the induction seen with 0.5 μM dexamethasone. PEPCK mRNA was induced to a level 9.3-fold higher than in controls when cells were co-incubated with cAMP and dexamethasone.

The rat proenkephalin gene is up-regulated by glucocorticoids and by elevations in cAMP levels and this up-regulation is synergistic when both drugs are added together in rat C6 glioma cells. Analysis of the proenkephalin promoter shows no functional GRE but several CREs. Reporter gene assays using the natural proenkephalin promoter show that, in contrast to whole cell studies, dexamethasone (10 μM) reduced CAT expression and inhibited the increased expression caused by forskolin (20 μM). Addition of a functional GRE in front of the proenkephalin promoter restored dexamethasone upregulation. This data suggests the presence of a functional GRE within the proenkephalin promoter and indicates one of the limitations of reporter gene assays [60].

Antagonism

Renal mesangial and vascular smooth muscle cells express inducible nitric oxide synthase (iNOS) in response to inflammatory cytokines such as interleukin (IL)-Iβ and agents that elevate cellular levels of cyclic AMP (cAMP). Bt_2cAMP (1 mM) induces iNOS gene transcription and mRNA half-life and this induction of iNOS protein and mRNA is inhibited in a dose-dependent manner by dexamethasone with a maximum at 1 μM. Furthermore, in these cells dexamethasone failed to inhibit IL-1β-stimulated iNOS synthesis although this is not case in pulmonary epithelial cells [61]. This suggests that dexamethasone acts at different levels, depending on the stimulus and cell used, to suppress iNOS induction [62].

Phosphoenolpyruvate carboxykinase (PEPCK) mRNA is increased 3-fold by the β-adrenergic agonist, isoprenaline (1 μM), and 8Br-cAMP (100 μM) in adipocytes. Dexamethasone (1 μM) decreased PEPCK mRNA by 80 % and also counteracted the inductive effects of isoprenaline and 8Br-cAMP with a half maximal inhibition at 1 nM. These actions appear to be mediated at the level of gene transcription [63]. Reporter gene assays using the PEPCK promoter show similar results with a 5-fold induction of luciferase activity with isoprenaline (1 μM) which is reduced by concomitant incubation with 1 μM dexamethasone. This is in contrast to the results seen in hepatocytes. The different effects of dexamethasone on PEPCK gene expression in liver and adipocytes are of particular interest as the PEPCK gene is a single copy gene under the regulation of a single promoter [64]. This suggests the requirement for other cell specific factors in mediating these drug effects on PEPCK gene expression.

The regulation of the obesity gene (ob) and its gene product leptin are tightly regulated both in humans and in rodent models. Experiments in cultured rat adipocytes shows that dexamethasone caused a dose-dependent 3-fold increase in leptin secretion which reached a maximum at 25 nM. This increase was preceded by a similar increase in ob gene expression. Conversely Bt_2cAMP (0.5 mM) and isoprenaline (10 μM) both cause a marked (up tp 85 %) reduction in both ob mRNA and leptin secretion in these cells [65]. Similarly the regulation of the human glucose-6-phosphate gene is controlled by both dexamethasone and intracellular levels of cAMP in H4IIE cells [66]. The Glucose-6-phosphate promoter, which contains no GRE, was activated by almost 40-fold by dexamethasone (1 μM) in these cells. Bt_2cAMP (500 μM) which alone had no effect on promoter activity suppressed the dexamethasone induction by 80 %.

Chromatin structure can markedly influence the response of a promoter to activation of the cAMP signalling pathway. Thus 8-Br cAMP synergises significantly with glucocorticoids in activating the transiently transfected mouse mammary tumour virus (MMTV) template. In contrast, 8-Br-cAMP is antagonistic to hormone-induced activation of the stably replicating MMTV template. Nuclear run-on

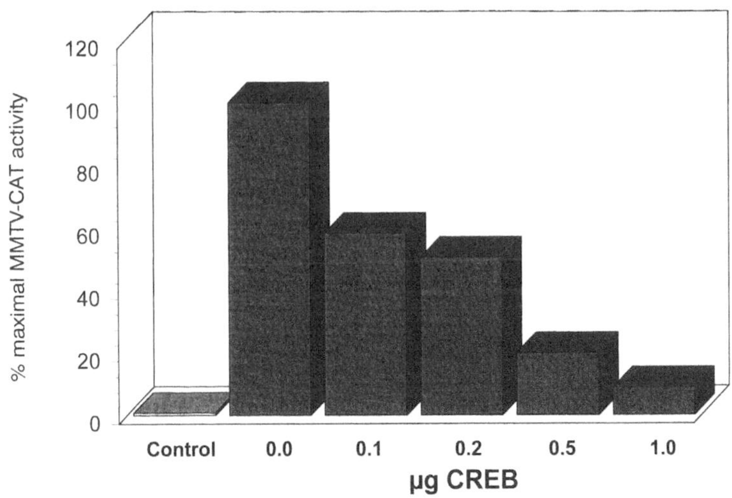

Fig. 5. Overexpression of CREB protein on GR- responsive gene transcription. Addition of increasing concentrations of recombinant CREB protein cells causes a dose dependent inhibition of dexamethasone-stimulated gene transcription as indicated by repression of mouse mammary virus (MMTV)-induced chloramphenicol acetyl transferase (CAT) activity in placental JEG-3 cells (calculated from data in ref. 45)

experiments demonstrate that this is a transcriptional effect on both hormone-induced transcription and on basal transcription. 8-Br cAMP does not inhibit GR DNA binding but inhibits GR-transcription initiation complex interactions [67].

Transcription of the glycocoprotein hormone alpha subunit gene is repressed by glucocorticoids in a cell and tissue type manner. However, mutation of the promoter sequences indicates that specific DNA binding to the alpha-subunit promoter is not important for repression. Inhibition by GR is only effective when the alpha-subunit promoter is activated by CREB, implicating CREB as the target for GR-mediated repression Reciprocally, overexpression of CREB interferes with GR-mediated transcriptional activation of MMTV (Fig. 5). This activity is not affected by the phosphorylation state of CREB. In these studies, despite the mutual cross-interference with activation of gene expression, GR and CREB do not appear to have a high affinity protein: protein interaction in vitro but may interact through a third protein or, more likely, may sequester a mutually required target protein [45].

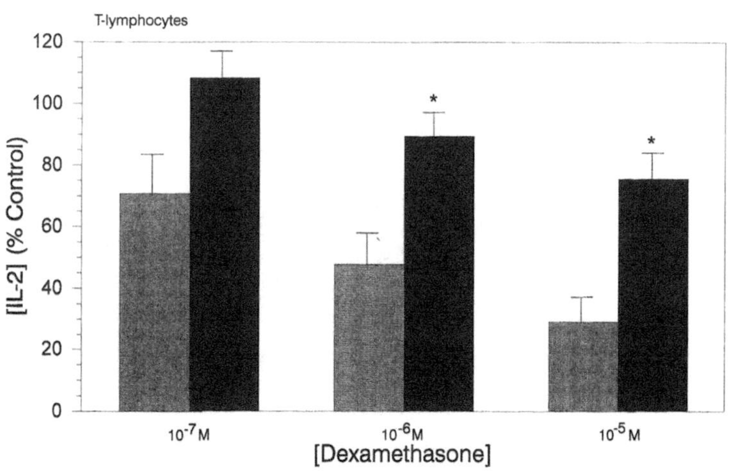

Fig. 6. The effect of vehicle (light bars) and salbutamol (0.1 mM) (dark bars) on the dose-dependent inhibition of IL-2 release from cultured PHA-stimulated human T-lymphocytes by 10 μM dexamethasone. The results are expressed as a percentage of the IL-2 release at zero dexamethasone concentration (*P<0.05)

In human and rat lung [46, 68], human lung epithelial cells and human T-cells [69, 70] the β_2-agonists, salbutamol and fenoterol, decrease the binding of GR to GRE although they have no effect on the affinity or number of glucocorticoid receptors. The effect of these β-agonists on GR phosphorylation status in these samples was not examined. Functionally, exposure to salbutamol (10^{-4}M) abrogated (70%) the inhibitory effect of dexamethasone (10 μM) on lectin-induced IL-2 release by CD4+ T-cells, with a significant shift of the concentration-response curve (Dr CJ Corrigan, personal communication; Fig. 6). In the lung epithelial cell line, A549, this inhibition of GRE binding by salbutamol is concentration-dependent, can be blocked by propranolol and is also seen following forskolin treatment. This effect appears to be due to an interaction between the GR and CREB, which was activated by very high concentrations of β_2-agonists (10^{-4}M). Further evidence of a direct interaction was the ability of excess unlabelled CRE oligonucleotide to directly compete with labelled GRE in the GR/GRE EMSA assay (IMA & DAS, unpublished observations). Furthermore the ability of GR to produce a Dnase 1 footprint within the MMTV-LTR was markedly reduced by the presence of salbutamol suggesting that this interaction directly inhibited the ability of GR to bind to its DNA binding site. Functionally this produced an impairment of GR mRNA regulation within A549 cells such that the dexamethasone-induced up-regulation of GR mRNA seen in these cells after 1 hr was attenuated by the presence of 1 μM salbutamol. Confirmation of the CREB/GR interaction was obtained using antisense oligonucleotides directed against CREB. Suppression of CREB synthesis prevented the reduction in GRE binding seen following salbutamol treatment (1 μM) in these cells (Fig. 7). By this mechanism, in these important cell types, high doses of inhaled β_2-agonists may inhibit the anti-inflammatory effects of endogenous glucocorticoids and exogenous corticosteroids used for asthma therapy [46].

Conclusion

Thus glucocorticoids and β_2-agonists may regulate gene transcription in a cell- and gene-specific manner at both the transcriptional and post-transcriptional level. For this transcription factor interaction to be of

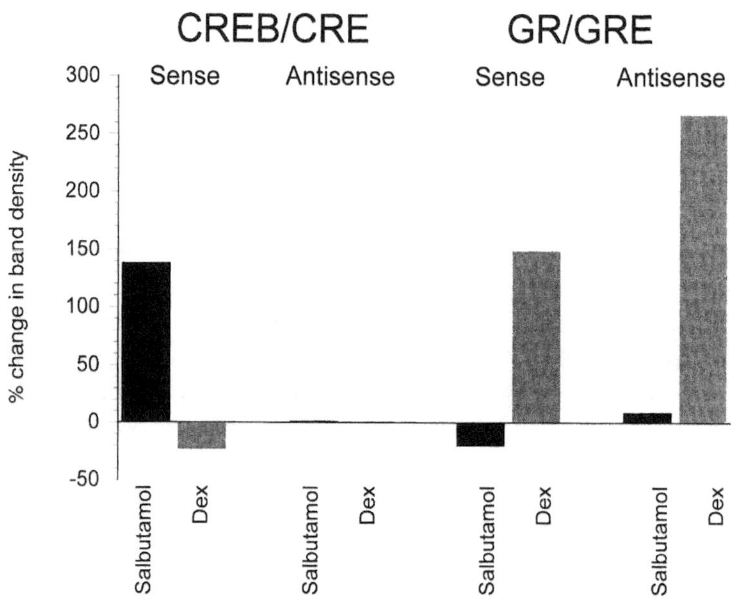

Fig. 7. The effect of incubation of A549 cells with a 10 μg specific sense or antisense CREB oligonucleotide for 72 hrs on CREB/CRE and GR/GRE binding following either salbutamol or dexamethasone treatment (both at 1 μM). The results are plotted as the % change in specific DNA binding and are the means of two separate experiments

importance in asthma, it must occur in a cell or cells which are key targets for steroids and which also express surface β_2-receptors and respond to β_2-agonist stimulation with elevation of cAMP. Many pulmonary cells express β_2-receptors [16, 71] and these same cells express GR [72]. Airway epithelial cells, T-lymphocytes and macrophages are target cells an which this effect may be of therapeutic relevance, particularly as all produce cytokines which may orchestrate or perpetuate the allergic inflammatory response [73].

Acknowledgements

We would like to thank The National Asthma Campaign, The Medical Research Council and Glaxo-Wellcome for sponsoring research in the authors laboratory.

References

1. Barnes PJ (1995) Inhaled glucocorticoids for asthma. N Engl J Med 332: 868–875
2. Munck A, Guyre PM, Holbrook NJ (1984) Physiological functions of glucocorticoids in stress and their relation to pharmacological actions. Endocrine Revs 5: 25–44
3. Truss M, Beato M (1993) Steroid hormone receptors: interaction with deoxyribo-nucleic acid and transcription factors. Endocrine Revs 14: 459–479
4. Truss M, Chalepakis G, Beato M (1992) Interplay of steroid hormone receptors and transcription factors on the mouse mammary tumour virus promoter. J Steroid Biochem Molec Biol 43: 365–378
5. Jonat C, Rahmsdorf HJ, Park K-K, Cato ACB, Gebel S, Ponta H, Herrlich P (1990) Antitumour promotion and antiinflammation: down-modulation of AP-1 (Fos/Jun) activity by glucocorticoid hormone. Cell 62: 1189–1204
6. Ray A, Prefontaine KE (1994) Physical association and functional antagonism between the p65 subunit of transcription factor NF-κB and the glucocorticoid receptor. Proc Nat Acad Sci (USA) 91: 752–756
7. Adcock IM, Brown CR, Gelder CM, Shirasaki H, Peters MJ, Barnes PJ (1995) Effects of glucocorticoids on transcription factor activation in human peripheral blood mononuclear cells. Am J Physiol 268: C331–C338
8. Adcock IM, Gelder CM, Shirasaki H, Yacoub M, Barnes PJ (1992) Effects of steroids on transcription factors in human lung. Am Rev Respir Dis 143: A834
9. Adcock IM, Shirasaki H, Gelder CM, Peters MJ, Brown CR, Barnes PJ (1994) The effects of glucocorticoids on phorbol ester and cytokine stimulated transcription factor activation in human lung. Life Sci 55: 1147–1153
10. Barnes PJ, Adcock IM (1993) Antiinflammatory actions of steroids: molecular mechanisms. Trends Pharmacol Sci 14: 436–441
11. Janknecht R, Hunter T (1996) A growing co-activator network. Nature 383: 22–23
12. Kamei Y, Xu L, Heinzel T, Torchia J, Kurokawa R, Gloss B, Lin S-C, Heyman RA, Rose DW, Glass CK, Rosenfeld MG (1996) A CBP integrator complex mediates transcriptional activation and AP-1 inhibition by nuclear receptors. Cell 85: 403–414
13. Chakravarti D, LaMorte VJ, Nelson MC, Nakajima T, Schulman IG, Juguilon H, Montminy M, Evans RM (1996) Role of CBP/P300 in nuclear receptor signalling. Nature 383: 99–103
14. Smith CL, Onate SA, Tsai M-J, O'Malley BW (1996) CREB binding protein acts synergistically with steroid receptor co-activator-1 to enhance steroid receptor-dependent transcription. Proc Natl Acad Sci USA 93: 8884–8888

15. Zhang X, Jeyakumar M, Bagchi MK (1996) Ligand-dependent cross-talk between steroid and thyroid receptors. J Biol Chem 271: 14825–14833
16. Barnes PJ, Basbaum CB, Nadel JA, Roberts JM (1982) Localization of beta-adrenoreceptors in mammalian lung by light microscopic autoradiography. Nature 299: 444–447
17. Barnes PJ (1995) Beta-adrenergic receptors and their regulation Am J Respir Crit Care Med 152: 838–860
18. Torphy TJ (1994) β-Adrenoceptors/cAMP and airway smooth muscle relaxation: challenges to the dogma. Trends Pharmacol Sci 15: 370–374
19. Kume H, Graziano MP, Kotlikoff MI (1992) Stimulatory and inhibitory regulation of calcium-activated potassium channels by guanine nucleotide-binding proteins. Proc Nat Acad Sci (USA) 89: 11051–11055
20. Yamamoto KK, Gonzalez GA, Biggs WH III, Montminy MR (1989) Phosphorylation-iduced binding and transcriptional efficacy of nuclear factor CREB. Nature 334: 494–498
21. Gonzalez GA, Montminy MR (1989) Cyclic AMP stimulates somatostatin gene transcription by phosphorylation of CREB at serine 133. Cell 59: 675–680
22. Sasaki K, Cripe TP, Koch SR, Andreone TL, Petersen DD, Beale EG, Granner DK (1984) Multihormonal regulation of phosphoenolpyruvate carboxykinase gene transcription. The dominant role of insulin. J Biol Chem 259: 15242–15251
23. Nigg EA, Hilz H, Eppenberger HM, Dutly F (1985) Rapid and reversible translocation of the catalytic subunit of cAMP-dependent protein kinase type II from the Golgi complex to the nucleus. EMBO J 4: 2801–2806
24. Kwok RPS, Lundblad JR, Chrivia JC, Richards JP, Bachinger HP, Brennan RG, Roberts SGE, Green MR, Goodman RH (1994) Nuclear protein CBP is a co-activator for the transcription factor CREB. Nature 370: 223–226
25. Kobierski LA, Chu H-M, Tan Y, Comb MJ (1991) cAMP-dependent regulation of proenkephalin by JunD and JunB: positive and negative effects of AP-1 proteins Proc Natl Acad Sci USA 88: 10222–10226
26. Masquilier D, Sassone-Corsi P (1992) Transcriptional cross-talk: nuclear factors CREM and CREB bind to AP-1 sites and inhibit activation by Jun. J Biol Chem 267: 22460–22466
27. Wu J, Dent P, Jelinek T, Wolfman A, Weber MJ, Sturgill TW (1993) Inhibition of the EGF-activated MAP kinase signallling pathway by adenosine 3',5'-monophosphate. Science 262: 1065–1069
28. Serkkola E, Hurme M (1993) Synergism between protein-kinase C and cAMP-dependent pathways in the expression of the interleukin-1β gene is mediated via the activator-protein-1 (AP-1) enhancer activity. Eur J Biochem 213: 243–249
29. Hai T, Curran T (1991) Cross family dimerisation of transcription factors

Fos/Jun and ATF/CREB alters DNA binding specificity. Proc Natl Acad Sci USA 88: 3720–3724
30. Lalli E, Sassone-Corsi P (1994) Signal transduction and gene regulation: the nuclear response to cAMP. J Biol Chem 269: 17359–17362
31. Collins S, Bouvier M, Bolanowski MA, Caron MG, Lefkowitz RJ (1989) cAMP stimulates transcription of the beta 2-adrenergic receptor gene in response to short term agonist exposure. Proc Natl Acad Sci USA 86: 4853–4857
32. Collins S, Altschmied J, Herbsman O, Caron MG, Mellon PL, Lefkowitz RJ (1990) A cAMP response element in the beta 2-adrenergic receptor gene confers transcriptional autoregulation by cAMP. J Biol Chem 265: 19330–19335
33. Hadcock JR, Malbon CC (1988) Regulation of beta-adrenergic receptors by "permissive" hormones: glucocorticoids increase steady-state levels of receptor mRNA. Proc Natl Acad Sci USA 85: 8415–8419
34. Mak JCW, Nishikawa M, Barnes PJ (1995) Glucocorticosteroids increase β_2-adrenergic receptor transcription in human lung. Am J Physiol 268: L41–L46
35. Nishikawa M, Mak JC, Shirasaki H, Barnes PJ (1993) Differential down-regulation of pulmonary beta 1- and beta 2-adrenocepter messenger RNA with prolonged in vivo infusion of isoprenaline. Eur J Pharmacol 247: 131–138
36. Davis AO, Lefkowitz RJ (1984) Regulation of β-adrenergic receptors by steriod hormones. Annu Rev Physiol 46: 119–130
37. Kobilka BK, Frielle T, Dohlman HG, Bolanowski MA, Dixon RAF, Keller P, Caron MG, Lefkowitz RJ (1987) Delineation of the intronless nature of the genes for the human and hamster β_2-adrenergic receptor and their putative promoter regions. J Biol Chem 262: 7321–7327
38. Malbon CC, Hadcock JR (1988) Evidence that glucocorticoid response elements in the 5'-noncoding region of the hamster beta 2-adrenergic receptor gene are obligate for glucocorticoid regulation of receptor mRNA levels. Biochem Biophys Res Commun 154: 676–681
39. Dooley DJ, Bittiger H, Reymann NC (1986) CGP 20712 A: a useful tool for quantitating β_1- and β_2-adrenoceptors. Eur J Pharmacol 130: 137–139
40. Mak JCW, Nishikawa M, Shirasaki H, Miyayasu K, Barnes PJ (1995) Protective effects of dexamethasone on isoproterenol-induced down-regulation of pulmonary β_2R. J Clin Invest 96: 99–106
41. Galant SP, Duriseti L, Underwood S, Insel PA (1978) Decreased beta-adrenergic receptors on polymorphonuclear leukocytes after adrenergic therapy. N Engl J Med 299: 933–936
42. Hauck RW, Bohm M, Gengenbach S, Sunder-Plassmann L, Fruhmann G, Erdmann E (1990) Beta 2-adrenoceptors in human lung and peripheral

mononuclear leukocytes of untreated and terbutaline-treated patients. Chest 98: 376–381
43. Schule R, Muller M, Otsuka-Murakami H, Renkawitz R (1988) Cooperativity of the glucocorticoid receptor and the CACCC-box binding factor. Nature 332: 87–90
44. Strahle U, Schmid W, Schutz G (1988) Synergistic action of the glucocorticoid receptor with transcription factors. EMBO J 7: 3389–3395
45. Stauber C, Altschmied J, Akerblom IE, Marron JL, Mellon PL (1992) Mutual cross-interference between glucocorticoid receptor and CREB inhibits transactivation in placental cells. New Biologist 4: 527–540
46. Peters MJ, Adcock IM, Brown CR, Barnes PJ (1995) β-Adrenoceptor agonists interfere with glucocorticoid receptor DNA binding in rat lung. Eur J Pharm (Mol Pharm) 289: 275–281
47. Drouin J, Charron J, Gagner JP, Jeannotte L, Nemer M, Plante RK, Wrange O (1987) Pro-opiomelanocortin gene: a model for negative regulation of transcription by glucocorticoids. J Cell Biochem 35: 293–304
48. Schüle R, Rangarajan P, Kliewer S, Ransome LJ, Bolado J, Yang N, Verma IM, Evans RM (1990) Functional antagonism between onco-protein c-jun and the glucocorticoid receptor. Cell 62: 1217–1226
49. Yang-Yen H-F, Chambard J-C, Sun Y-L, Smeal T, Schmidt TJ, Drouin J, Karin M (1990) Transcriptional interference between c-Jun and the glucocorticoid receptor: Mutual inhibition of DNA binding due to direct protein-protein interaction. Cell 62: 1205–1215
50. Mukaida N, Morita M, Ishikawa Y, Rice N, Okamoto S, Kasahari T, Matsushima K (1994) Novel mechanism of glucocorticoid-mediated gene repression. Nuclear factor kappa B is the target for glucocorticoid-mediated interleukin-8 gene repression. J Biol Chem 269: 13289–13295
51. Newton R, Kuitert LM, Bergmann M, Adcock IM, Barnes PJ (1997) Evidence for involvement of NF-xB in the transcriptional control of cox-2 gene expression by IL-1_{β}. Biochem Biophys Res Comm 237: 46–50
52. Scarceriaux V, Pelaprat D, Forgez P, Lhiaubert AM, Rostene W (1995) Effects of dexamethasone and forskolin on neurotensin production in rat hypothalamic cultures. Endocrinology 136: 2554–2560
53. Kathju S, Heaton JH, Bruzdzinski CJ, Gelehrter TD (1994) Synergistic induction of tissue-type plasminogen activator gene expression by glucocorticoids and cyclic nucleotides in rat HTC hepatoma cells. Endocrinology 135: 1195–1204
54. Hinko A, Soloff MS (1993) Up-regulation of oxytocin receptors in rabbit amnion by glucocorticoids: potentiation by cyclic adenosine 3',5'-monophosphate. Endocrinology 133: 1511–1519
55. Michel MC, Knapp J, Ratjen H (1994) Sensitisation by dexamethasone of lymphocyte cyclic AMP formation: evidence for increased function of the adenylyl cyclase catalyst. Br J Pharmacol 113: 240–246

56. Liu J-L, Papachristou DN, Patel YC (1994) Glucocorticoids activate somatostatin gene transcription through cooperative interaction with the cyclic AMP signalling pathway. Biochem J 301: 863–869
57. Dong Y, Aronsson M, Gustaffson J-A, Okret S (1989) The mechanism of cAMP-induced glucocorticoid receptor expression: Correlation to cellular glucocorticoid response. J Biol Chem 264: 13679–13683
58. Nordeen SK, Moyer ML, Bona BJ (1994) The coupling of multiple signal transduction pathways with steroid response mechanisms. Endocrinology 134: 1723–1732
59. Imai E, Miner JN, Mitchell JA, Yamamoto KR, Granner DK (1993) Glucocorticoid receptor-cAMP response element-binding protein interaction and the response of the phosphoenolpyruvate carboxykinase gene to glucocorticoids. J Biol Chem 268: 5353–5356
60. Jenab S, Inturrisi CE (1995) Proenkephalin gene expression: interaction of glucocorticoid and cAMP regulatory elements. Biochem Biophys Res Comm 210: 589–599
61. Newton R, Kuitert LM, Barnes PJ, Adcock IM (1995) Stimulation of COX-2 message by cytokines of phorbol ester is preceded by a massive and rapid induction of NF-κB binding activity. Am J Resp Crit Care Med 151: A165
62. Kunz D, Walker G, Pfeilschifter J (1994) Dexamethasone differentially affects interleukin 1β- and cAMP-induced nitric oxide synthase mRNA expression in renal mesangial cells. Biochem J 304: 337–340
63. Franckhauser S, Antras-Ferry J, Robin P, Robin D, Granner DK, Forest C et al (1995) Expression of the phosphoenolpyruvate carboxykinase gene in 3T3-F442A adipose cells: opposite effects of dexamethasone and isoprenaline on transcription. Biochem J 305: 65–71
64. Beale EG, Chrapkiewicz NB, Scoble HA, Metz RJ, Quick DP, Noble RL, Donelson JE, Biemann K, Granner DK (1985) Rat hepatic cytosolic phosphoenolpyruvate carboxykinase (GTP). Structures of the protein, messenger RNA, and gene. J Biol Chem 260: 10748-60
65. Slieker LJ, Sloop KW, Surface PL, Kriauciunas A, LaQuier F, Manetta J, Bue-Valleskey J, Stephens TW (1996) Regulation of *ob* mRNA and protein by glucocorticoids and cAMP. J Biol Chem 271: 5301–5304
66. Schmoll D, Allan BB, Burchall A (1996) Cloning and sequencing of the 5′ region of the human glucose-6-phosphate gene: transcriptional regulation by cAMP, insulin and glucocorticoids in H4IIE cells. FEBS Letts 383: 63–66
67. Pennie WD, Hager GL, Smith CL (1995) Nucleoprotein structure influences the response of the mouse mammary tumor virus promoter to activation of the cyclic AMP signalling pathway. Mol Cell Biol 15: 2125–2134
68. Peters MJ, Adcock IM, Brown CR, Barnes PJ (1993) β-Agonist inhibition of steroid-receptor DNA binding activity in human lung. Am Rev Respir Dis 147: A772

69. Stevens DA, Barnes PJ, Adcock IM (1995) β-Agonists inhibit DNA binding of glucocorticoid receptors in human pulmonary and bronchial epithelial cells. Am J Respir Crit Care Med 151: A195
70. Adcock IM, Peters MJ, Kwon OJ, Corrigan G, Barnes PJ (1994) Glucocorticoid receptor interactions with cAMP response element binding protein (CREB) in specific target cells in the lung. Am J Respir Crit Care Med 149: A1026
71. Carstairs JR, Nimmo AJ, Barnes PJ (1985) Autoradiographic visualization of beta-adrenoreceptor subtypes in human lung. Am Rev Respir Dis 132: 541–547
72. Adcock IM, Gilbey T, Gelder CM, Chung KF, Barnes PJ (1996) Glucocorticoid receptor localisation in normal and asthmatic lung. Am J Respir Crit Care Med 154: 771–782
73. Arai K, Lee F, Miyajima A, Miyatake S, Arai N, Yokota T (1990) Cytokines: coordinators of immune and inflammatory responses. Annu Rev Biochem 59: 783–836

Correspondence: Dr. Ian M. Adcock, Department of Thoracic Medicine, Imperial College School of Medicine at NHLI, Dovehouse Street, London SW3 6LY, U. K.

Discussion

Dr. Block: Thank you very much for this very interesting data, which I think contained a number of aspects that need to be discussed.

Dr. Greening: A lot of fascinating stuff in that talk. In your last slide you appeared to show a clear difference between one long-acting beta-2 agonist and one short-acting beta-2 agonist. If as a simple clinician I look at the studies and say beta agonists are bad, I am only possibly persuaded about formoterol and not persuaded by the studies looking at other short-acting beta-2 agonists. Have you seen differences between the different short-acting beta-2 agonists in terms of dose-response relationships and doses at which there might be an interaction?

Dr. Adcock: Yes. Basically, most of the experiments which were performed by David Stevens in our lab, showed that fenoterol is far more inhibitory to the effects of dexamethasone in A549 cells and peripheral blood mononuclear cells than salbutamol. Although salbutamol causes a small rightward shift in the dexamethasone dose-response curve, this is not significant over the whole dose range and is probably of little functional effect. But clearly, fenoterol in the lower doses showed an enhancement of the ability of steroids to inhibit GM-CSF release. So I would agree that the clinical problems seen with fenoterol are probably related to the drug being a full agonist rather than a class effect since most clinically used ß-agonists are partial agonists. We've also looked at the $ß_1$ and $ß_2$-selective drug isoprenalinc. The data here is confusing but not too dissimilar from that seen with fenoterol.

Dr. Collins: A question that also related to the last slide. So what was the dose of the compounds?

Dr. Adcock: The fenoterol dose was 10^{-5} M and that for salbutamol was 10^{-6} M.

Dr. Ulmer: Thank you for this excellent paper. I have a problem. When you give glucocorticosteroids, how long does it need for all these mechanisms until the expression of new beta-receptors takes place?

Dr. Adcock: The message seems to be induced, at least in our hands, within the first two hours. Looking at binding studies, you're seeing some induction by eight hours, and at twenty-four hours we had peak induction.

Dr. Ulmer: This is relatively long, because, when we treat a patient in an asthmatic attack with water-soluble glucocorticosteroids, they seem to work after five minutes.

Dr. Adcock: Maybe because with glucocorticoids you're blocking the activity of a whole range of other mediators. Probably the most important mechanism of steroid action is not by the induction of various genes. It's by inhibition of mediators and their effects. And this can occur much quicker than the synthesis of new beta-2-receptors.

Dr. Ulmer: Are there are some other mechanisms which could be important in this context?

Dr. Adcock: It seems that is various other beta-agonists can also phosphorylate the glucocorticoid receptor. And at present no functional effects of that are known.

Dr. Ulmer: How long does it take for phosphorylation?

Dr. Adcock: That's the most immediate in the cell lines.

Dr. Ulmer: So beta-agonists work very short?

Dr. Adcock: Yes.

Dr. Ulmer: But glucocorticosteroids sometimes have a longer-acting effect?

Dr. Adcock: The ß-agonists act in the short term by causing smooth muscle relaxation by a mechanism that either involves cyclic AMP or, at least in our hands, probably by a non-cyclic AMP mechanism possibly by a direct interaction with maxi-K channels. This effect causes cell hyperpolarization and consequently smooth muscle relaxation within minutes of drug treatment. Most steroid effects occur over a much longer time course and are due to inhibition of chronic inflammatory events via effects on gene transcription. Generally steroids do not act immediately, although there are recent reports of non-genomic effects of steroids acting mainly on the membranes of neural cells. These effects have not been investigated within the lung to my knowledge. The normal homeostatic effect of steroids and their clinical actions are both to suppress inflammatory stimuli over a period of time. This suppression of the chronic inflammatory mechanisms underlying asthma is the important mechanism of steroid action. For this reason it is important that patients are maintained on the lowest dose of steroids possible once inflammation is brought under control with ß-agonists used to control breakthrough symptoms. Both classes of drugs are very good and have an important role to play clinically in the treatment of asthma.

Dr. Ulmer: How about preventing down-regulation? In our unit we had many hundreds of patients whom we treated continuously with beta-2 sympathicomimetics for more than 10 years. These were very sick patients but they could be maintained with a very small dose of glucocorticoids and clinically there was no downregulation.

Dr. Adcock: The EC50 that we found for glucocorticoids in a cell culture for inducing beta-2 receptor protein is in the region of 10^{-9} M, which is a level of steroid you find circulating within the blood. It's still reasonable to suggest that even with low doses you may actually prevent down-regulation. Studying cell cultures, we can modulate quite dramatically the amounts of drugs within our test system from zero to very high doses (10^{-4} M), which you can't do in a patient.

Formoterol, a new long-acting β_2-agonist

*G. Anderson**

Former address: Ciba-Geigy Limited, Basel, Switzerland
Present address: Department of Pharmacology,
University of Melbourne, Australia

Formoterol is a long acting, fast onset of action bronchodilator which is inreasingly widly used for the treatment of reversible airflow obstruction. Extensive clinical trials have demonstrated that formoterol produces bronchodilation lasting 12 hours with a very rapid onset of action (2–3 min.). These properties support the use of formoterol in clinical situations where sustained relief or prophylaxis of airflow obstruction is warranted, for example in moderate or severe asthmatics and those suffering from nocturnal asthma. While the clinical advantages of formoterol over more familiar drugs such as salbutamol and terbutaline have been relatively easy to demonstrate understanding exactly why Formoterol has these properties has required extensive molecular pharmacology and biophysical analysis.

The receptor pharmacology of formoterol has been very well characterised. Formoterol was developed from earlier phenylethanolamine precursors by systematically optimizing the molecule for three parameters 1) β_2 adrenoceptor selectivity 2) receptor affinity (potency) and 3) receptor efficacy (efficiency of stimulating signal transduction).

This research lead to the identification of formoterol as an extremely

---

* The author apologizes for not being able to furnish a full manuscript.

β_2 adrenoceptor selective, highly potent and very efficient agonist. Even in the earliest stages of development it was clear that formoterol also showed a superior duration of action compared to salbutamol.

However it was not until the discovery that formoterol, like salbutamol, is difficult to wash free from human bronchi and that formoterol causes "reassertion relaxation" that research began to focus on the biophysical properties of the molecule.

Detailed biophysical analysis strongly suggests that a fraction of the inhaled dose of formoterol enters the outer cell membrane phospholipid where it forms a "micro-depot" while the majority gains rapid access to β_2 adrenoceptors.

Careful analysis strongly suggests that the long duration of action of formoterol can not be due to interactions with the putative β_2-adrenoceptors exosite. Indeed careful study of close molecular analogies of salmeterol strongly suggests that such an exosite does not exist.

Collectively, the data currently available suggests that the properties of all long acting β_2-agonists can only be understood by analysis of receptor interactions which dictate the nature of the bronchodilator response and drug biophysics which determine tissue and cellular distribution and have an impact on onset and duration. These data may have important implications for optimizing patient therapy.

Correspondence: Dr. Gary Anderson, Department of Pharmacology, University of Melbourne, Parkville, Victoria 3052, Australia.

Discussion

The discussion to this lecture was held in combination with that of the following lecture.

Development of the long-acting β_2-agonist, salmeterol

M. Johnson

Glaxo Wellcome Research and Development, U.K.

Summary

The objective of developing a drug with therapeutically significant, sustained bronchodilator activity for the treatment of reversible airways obstruction, when administered by the inhaled route, has been achieved in the new generation of long-acting β_2-agonists, represented by salmeterol. As a result of potent and prolonged activation of β_2-adrenoceptors in airways smooth muscle, salmeterol produces bronchodilation for at least 12 h. This pharmacological activity arises from the novel mechanism of action of salmeterol, whereby as a direct consequence of the design features of the molecule, it is localised in a specific exo-site domain of the β_2-receptor protein, from where it can continuously stimulate the active site of the receptor.

Introduction

Bronchial asthma is now recognised as a complex multifactorial disease characterised by episodic bronchoconstriction, airway hyper-reactivity, inflammation, and muco-cililary abnormalities [1]. For many years, adrenaline was used as a bronchodilator for the treatment of asthma, but the discovery of α- and β-adrenoceptors opened up the possibility of developing a more β-selective compound to avoid some of the side effects of adrenaline. Isoprenaline was the first of such compounds, and as a highly β-selective adrenoceptor agonist, proved to be a significant advance over adrenaline in the treatment of airways constriction [2]. However, although an effective bronchodilator, its use was also associated with unacceptable extra-pulmonary side effects. It was the timely β-receptor subclassification proposed by Lands and his colleagues [3] that made possible the development of agonists selective for β_2-adrenoceptors, which produced marked bronchodilation without the concomitant tachycardia associated with the earlier compounds. The prototype β_2-adrenoceptor agonist was salbutamol (Ventolin™) showing a > 500-fold separation in activity at β_2 over β_1 receptors [4]. One clear shortcoming of the potent, selective β_2-adrenoceptor agonists developed in the late 1960's and 1970's, and exemplified by salbutamol, terbutaline and fenoterol, is their duration of action. In each case, the bronchodilator activity resulting from a single administration of the drug, whether by inhalation or by mouth, has no more than 4–6 h duration, and this is clearly inadequate for protection from bronchospasm through the night, or to provide convenient maintenance therapy for the asthmatic patient.

The challenge was to develop a drug which would be effective for >12 h. In the early 1980's, work in a number of pharmaceutical companies was underway with the target of developing an inherently long-acting drug, that would be suitable for twice-a-day treatment. A prolonged duration of action of systemically administered drugs can be achieved with an appropriate pharmacokinetic profile, ie, resistance to metabolism and low plasma clearance. Indeed, clenbuterol is such a compound, and does have a prolonged duration of action after oral administration. Alternatively, a relatively labile drug may be formulated in such a way as to delay systemic release, and salbutamol has been prepared as a delayed release formulation [5]. Finally, a drug may be prepared as a pro-drug, ie; a drug which is inactive in its own right, but which is slowly metabolised to an active entity, and both bitolterol [6] and bambuterol [7], terbutaline prodrugs, have achieved an extended duration of action. The main problem with orally administered β_2-agonists is their side-effect liability, with physiological tremor and tachycardia being particular problems. It is for this reason that a different approach to an inherently long-acting β_2-agonist was required.

Design of a long-acting β_2-agonist

A research programme was initiated at Glaxo Group Research in 1980, with the concept that it would be possible to design a chemical entity which would have a long duration of action by virtue of increased specific binding in the vicinity of the β-adrenoceptor. The new molecule would have two major sites of interaction; one at the active site of the β-receptor and the other at a nearby, specific site, possibly in an adjacent non-polar region of the cell membrane or in a hydrophobic domain of the receptor protein [8]. Such a molecule would persist at its additional binding site (s) through an anchoring mechanism, while the functional centre repeatedly stimulated the active site of the receptor. If successful, given binding of sufficient affinity, the new β-agonist would therefore be retained at its site of action on the β_2-adrenoceptor protein and the resulting drug-receptor complex that catalyses the cellular response would, provided it retained its efficacy, be effective for longer.

The chemical rationale adopted was to introduce large, lipophilic N-substitutents into saligenin ethanolamines, in an attempt to engage any exo-receptor binding sites, as well as to increase potency and selectivity [8]. Saligenins were selected as the molecular configuration of the new compound, based on the fact that low toxicity was associated with this structural type, from the experience with salbutamol, and that well-defined synthetic methods already existed for these compounds.

There was evidence to support the strategy of incorporating lipophilic, bulky substituents into a saligenin to obtain long-acting compounds (Table 1). Salmefamol, which contains a branched phenylethyl substituent was found to be longer acting (6 h) than salbutamol as a bronchodilator in man [9]. Comparison of calculated log P values (a measure of lipophilicity) revealed that salmefamol had a log P of 1.68 compared with 0.66 for salbutamol. The enhanced duration of action observed was sufficiently encouraging for other spacer groups between the N-atom and the terminal aryl ring to be examined. One such group was the hexyloxyethyl unit. Introduction of this spacer into the saligenin

Table 1. Substitution of spacer groups between (N) and terminal aryl ring

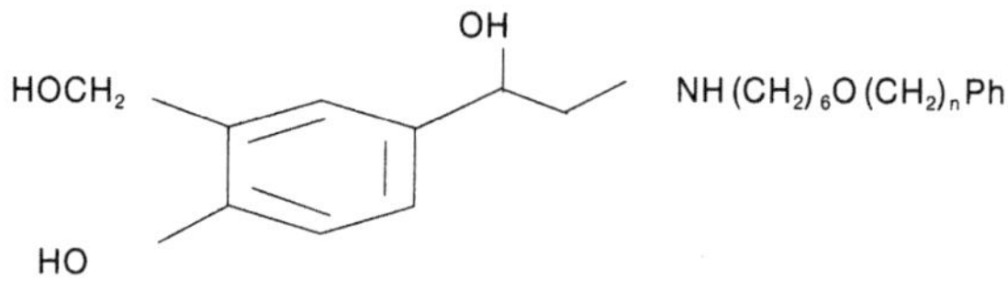

n	β_2-Potency* (Isoprenaline = 1)	Duration of Action* (min)	Log P
Salbutamol	2.0	3.7	0.66
Salmefamol	2.7	7.3	1.68
2	0.5	189	2.80
3	1.2	> 400	3.35
4 (Salmeterol)	0.9	> 420 – > 720	3.88

*Electrically-stimulated guinea-pig trachea preparation

afforded a compound which was equipotent with isoprenaline, but with a considerably longer duration of action (Table 1). The calculated log P of this compound was 2.8. Sequential extension of the chain gave further analogues with comparable potencies but, more importantly, with enhanced durations of action (Table 1).

A considerable amount of structure-activity (SAR) investigation was carried out around the series. In Table 2, the effect of modifying the length of the alkyl functionality adjacent to the side-chain ether group is shown. Two observations can be made from this data. Firstly, to maintain potency, (*m*) should equal 5 or 6 carbon atoms and (*n*) should be 2–4 carbon atoms [10]. Secondly, to obtaun a long duration of action, the calculated log P value should be within the range 3.3–4.5 [10]. Log P values <3.3 invariably resulted in short-acting compounds in vitro. These compound variants also indicated the importance of the position of the 0 atom in the side chain. For example, with the oxygen placed towards the nitrogen, the duration of action was only 2.7 min; when the 0 atom was positioned close to the terminal phenyl ring, again the duration of action was limited to <50 min [10]. Optimal activity

Table 2. Structure-activity relationships in the saligenin ethanolamine series

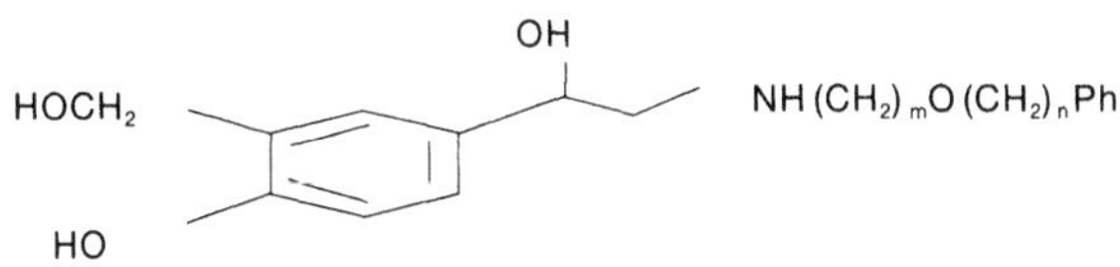

m	n	Log P	β_2-Potency (Isoprenaline = 1)	Duration of Action (Min)
2	8	3.88		2.7
4	3	2.30	100.0	6.8
4	4	2.83	17.1	20.5
4	5	3.30	10.5	> 30.0
4	6	3.88	6.5	> 60.0
5	2	2.30	1.2	5.0
5	3	2.83	3.6	> 14.0
5	4	3.35	0.5	> 30.0
5	5	3.88	1.4	> 400.0
6	1	2.30	10.5	6.5
6	2	2.83	1.1	10.7
6	3	3.35	2.4	> 35.0
6 (Salmeterol)	4	3.88	0.9	> 720.0
6	5	4.41	5.6	> 300.0
6	6	4.08	7.8	290.0
7	3	3.88	8.8	> 300.0
8	2	3.88		> 30.0
9	1	3.88		47.6

(duration of action >720 min) appeared with a side chain skeleton comprising 11 atoms, in a $(CH_2)_6 0$ $(CH_2)_4$ configuration, together with a terminal phenyl group (Fig. 1). This compound is salmeterol, with a calculated log P of 3.88.

In summary, from structure-acitivity relationship in a series of N-aralkyloxyalkyl analogues of salbutamol, it emerged that there were several factors which determined duration of action as β-agonists; the overall lipophilicity of the molecule and both the length of the side chain, and the presence and position of an 0 atom. As the size of the side

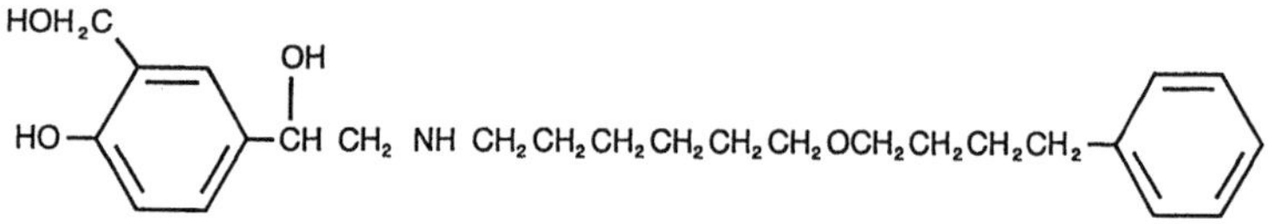

Fig. 1. Structure of the salmeterol molecule

chain was increased, there was a prolongation in the activity of the β-agonist molecules in relaxing airways smooth muscle. It was also clear that although the associated increase in lipophilicity was important, it was not the only critical factor, since further increases in chain length and lipophilicity resulted in a decrease in duration of action. Salmeterol in the form of the hydroxynaphthoate salt (Serevent™) was selected for development by Glaxo in 1981.

The salmeterol molecule

The molecular structure of a β-adrenoceptor agonist determines its physicochemical properties. The salmeterol molecule is 25 Å compared with 11 Å for salbutamol. It is > 10,000 times more lipophilic than salbutamol, with an octanol-water partition coefficient of 7600 and a partition coefficient in biological membranes of 22,500 [11]. The lipophilicity of the β-agonist determines the degree of partitioning into the cell membrane and subsequent diffusion kinetics in interacting with the β-adrenoceptor. In the case of salbutamol, which is hydrophilic in nature, the molecule remains in the extracellular aqueous compartment. The drug accesses the active site of the β-adrenoceptor directly, but rapidly re-equilibrates with the aqueous phase and therefore its residency time at the active site is limited and its duration of action is short. The use of low-angle neutron diffraction techniques to study the interaction of salmeterol with the cell membrane, has indicated that as a result of its lipophilic properties, salmeterol partitions rapidly (< 1 min) into the outer phospholipid monolayer by a factor approaching 30,000:1 [11]. Molecular modelling suggests that the orientation is such that the saligenin moiety is the same plane as the polar head groups, with the side-chain in close association with the hydrophobic tails of the phospholipids. It is of interest that the 17 Å side chain of salmeterol, which was found to be optimal for duration of action, is the same as the depth of the phospholipid monolayer. There is no evidence that salmeterol "flip-flops" from the outer to the inner monolayers of the surface phospholipids, but instead the molecule diffuses laterally to approach the active site of the β-adrenoceptor through the membrane [12]. This translocation process appears to be slow (> 30 min). Although salmeterol less readily re-equilibrates with the extracellular aqueous phase, on washing, it does dissociate from membrances with a half life of approximately 30 min [11], suggesting that there is another mechanism involved in the long duration of action (> 7 h) of the compound.

Salmeterol interaction with the β-adrenoceptor

Site-directed mutagenesis has been used to identify regions of the β_2-adrenoceptor protein important for ligand and G-protein coupling [13]. It is generally agreed that there are residues of critical importance with respect to agonist binding, namely the aspartate (Asp)-residue 113 (counted from the extracellular or N-terminus end) of the third domain, two serine (Ser) residues, 204 and 207, which are both on the fifth domain and two phenylalanines (Phe), 259 and 290, on the sixth domain [14]. Thus, a model has emerged for the agonist binding site of the β_2-adrenoceptor in which the ligand is bound within the hydrophobic core of the protein, intercalated among the transmembrane helices, and anchored by specific molecular interactions between amino acid residues in the receptor and functional groups on the ligand [15]. Asp binds to the nitrogen of the β-adrenoceptor agonist molecule, while the two Ser residues interact with the hydroxyl groups on the phenyl ring.

β-receptor modelling

At Glaxo Group Research a model of the β_2-receptor was constructed using bovine opsin as an intermediary to align bacteriorhodopsin and the β_2-receptor [16]. The important aspect of the modelling work was to examine the potential modes of binding of salmeterol at the receptor. Assuming salmeterol binds to the same funcional groups at the agonist binding site, the long flexible – $(CH_2)_6O(CH_2)_4Ph$ chain can in principle, fit in the receptor in three orientations [16]. In these orientations, there are serine or threonine residues in proximity of the ether oxygen linkage that could form hydrogen bonds ($^{Thr}110$, $^{Ser}120$ and $^{Ser}165$ for "up", "down" and "membrane" orientations, respectively). If hydrogen bonding with the side-chain ether oxygen is an important component in the binding of salmeterol at the receptor, then the SAR observed can be rationalised. Should (m) or (n) fall outside the optimum range presumably the ether oxygen cannot then form an efficient hydrogen bond with the appropriate amino acid.

The "up" orientation may be the least likely, since in this position the highly lipophilic side chain of salmeterol would be located in regions of the receptor containing hydrophilic amino acids. With regard to the membrane orientation, Rhodes et al. [11] have shown that salmeterol is avidly absorbed into membrances and that it accesses the active site of the receptor via the lipid bilayer. If the tail remains within the membrane, thus anchoring the molecule, is the bulk lipid of the membrane, in effect, an additional binding site? This hypothetical mode of binding would explain why structurally similar compounds to salmeterol, but with lower log P values, are not long acting. These compounds cannot approach the active site in the same way since their lower lipophilicity precludes initial membrane uptake. Such compounds must access the receptor directly from the extra-cellular fluid and it is possible that then they cannot adopt the membrane orientation of salmeterol. However, functional evidence indicates that the long duration of action of salmeterol may be unique to β_2-adrenoceptor-containing tissues [17]. This suggests that the "down" orientation, where the salmeterol molecule is located within the receptor protein structure, but with the side chain in a region of hydrophobic amino acids, may be the preferred conformation. Clearly, this interpretation of the mode of salmeterol binding was speculative and could only be confirmed by further experimentation.

Analysis of the β-agonist binding kinetics indicates [18] that while the binding of salbutamol and other β-agonists to lung membranes is competitive in nature, and the molecules readily dissociate from their binding sites ($T^1/_2$, 10 min), the binding kinetics of salmeterol are non-competitive, and the dissociation rate is very slow ($T^1/_2$ >300 min). This difference in binding characteristics is reflected in the comparative pharmacological activity of salmeterol. Salmeterol was originally identified as being extremely long-acting as a β_2-adrenoceptor agonist in isolated airway preparations, such as the guinea pig trachea and human bronchus, where after a single exposure of the tissue to the agonist, even continuous washing for periods in excess of 10 h failed to cause any decline in the β_2-adrenoceptor agonist activity [19]. Such persistence of action, although clearly β-receptor mediated, does not result from irreversible binding to the active site of the β_2-adrenoceptor itself, since rapid and complete reversal of the effects of salmeterol can be achieved by relatively low concentrations of β-adrenoceptor blocking drugs, such as propranolol and sotalol, indicating a competitive interaction with the β-receptor. An important and interesting observation is, however, that following washout of the β-adrenoceptor blocking drug, and without administration of further salmeterol, the β_2-agonist relaxant effects are reasserted and this pattern of reversal and reassertion can be repeated several times [20]. Similarly, while salmeterol had no effect in airways preparations, in the presence of a β-blocker, it exerts normal relaxant activity many hours later, following termination of the antagonist administration [20]. None of these properties are demonstrated by other β-agonists. Taken together, the data suggests that salmeterol persists in tissues, but in a specific manner that enables the molecule to interact freely and reversibly with the active site of the β-adrenoceptor. Work on a series of human cloned β-receptor subtypes in transfected cells, and in intact tissue, shows salmeterol to be both long-acting and to posses the phenomenon of reassertion of activity after β-blocker reversal only at β_2 receptors [21]. Finally, if the salmeterol sidechain is added to a β-blocker such as the β_1-selective antagonist, atenolol, which has an approximately 100-fold selectivity for β_1 over β_2 receptors, the hybrid molecule becomes a long-acting, β_2-selective compound [22]. This experiment has been repeated with a number of different types of β-receptor antagonists. Lipophilicity alone, as suggested by Anderson et al. [23], cannot, therefore, explain the duration of action of the molecule, salmeterol. Instead, the data suggest that the nature of the side chain in some way evokes a specific interaction with β_2-adrenoceptors.

In order to rationalise the experimental findings that the receptor binding of salmeterol is only slowly reversible and non-competitive, whereas functional responses to the molecule are both fully reversible and competitive, the "exo-site" hypothesis was proposed [24]. The original concept [8] was that the long-side chain of the molecule interacted with a nonpolar region in the cell membrane, the "exo-site", in the vicinity of the β-receptor. High affinity binding of the side-chain to the exo-site then allowed the saligenin head to repeatedly activate the receptor, enabling salmeterol to be long-acting without causing desensitization or tachyphylaxis. From the molecular modelling studies [16], it has been predicted that there is a preferred "down" conformation of the molecule in the receptor protein, whereby the saligenin head binds to the active site in an analogous position to that of salbutamol, and the long, flexible side-chain is located deep into a hydrophobic core domain of the receptor. The latter may then represent the specific "exo-site" for salmeterol, an integral part of the β_2-adrenoceptor protein itself:

The wealth of circumstantial evidences therefore supports the existence of the exo-site, but clear evidence for its location has, until recently, been absent. However, work involving the use of hybrid forms of the β_2-adrenoceptor [25] has cast considerable light on this question. These studies involved the substitution of amino acid sequences of the β_2-adrenoceptor by the corresponding sequence from the β_1-adrenoceptor by site-directed mutagenesis. They showed that it was possible to replace a discrete length of the fourth transmembrane domain of the β_2-adrenoceptor (specifically, residues 149–158, believed to be associated with exosite binding, see Fig. 2) with the corresponding section of the β_1-adrenoceptor, while maintaining the affinity of salmeterol for the resulting hybrid receptor. However, significantly, this modification resulted in a decreased persistence of agonist activity after washout. Even more significantly, when the corresponding β_1-adrenoceptor hybrid was constructed with the same key amino acids (methionine, leucine, isoleucine, isoleucine, valine) from the β_2-adrenoceptor, this resulted in markedly enhanced persistence of salmeterol activity [26].

The mechanism of action of salmeterol therefore involves the interaction of the side chain of the salmeterol with an auxiliary binding site (exo-site), a domain of hydrophobic amino acids within the fourth domain of the β_2-adrenoceptor (Fig. 2). When the side chain is in association with the exo-site, the molecule is prevented from dissociating

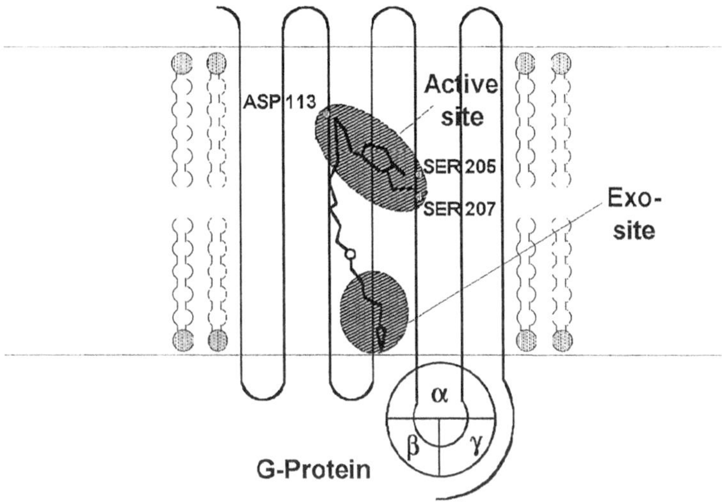

Fig. 2. The mechanism of action of salmeterol. The salmeterol molecule is illustrated with the saligenin head interacting with the active site of the β_2-adrenoceptor and with the longipophilic side chain bound to the exo-site, a series of hydrophobic aminoacids in the terminal area of the fourth domain

from the β_2-adrenoceptor, but the saligenin head can freely engage and disengage the active site (Fig. 2) by the Charnière (hinge) principle [27], flexion being about the 0 atom in the side-chain, the position of which the SAR showed to be critical for duration of action.

Pharmacology of salmeterol

The novel mechanism of action of salmeterol, which is not shared by other β-agonists, provides the drug with a unique profile of pharmacological activity. The first example of this is in the β-adrenoceptor selectivity of the molecule, which is an important factor in the safety of the β-agonists.

β_2-adrenoceptor selectivity

The aim of bronchodilator therapy should be to produce an optimal airways response, with minimal systemic adverse effects. The latter may be divided into those which are β_2-adrenoceptor mediated and include skeletal muscle tremor, hypokalaemia and ECG changes, and those such as heart rate which appear to be the result of direct stimulation of both β_1- and β_2-adrenoceptors [28].

β-adrenoceptors have now been further sub-classified into at least three distinct groups – β_1, β_2 and β_3 [29]. At β_2-adrenoceptors in airways smooth muscle, salmeterol is ca. 8-fold more potent than isoprenaline and significantly more potent than salbutamol [30]. In contrast, at cardiac β_1-adrenoceptors, although all β_2-agonists are less potent than isoprenaline, this ranges from 20-fold less for fenoterol (Table 3) to >10,000-fold less for salmeterol [30]. Salbutamol and salmeterol also have low potency at β_3-adrenoceptors, while fenoterol and formoterol are only 15- and 50-fold less potent than isoprenaline [30]. Fenoterol appears to exhibit the lowest selectivity compared with isoprenaline and salmeterol is the most functionally selective β_2-adrenoceptor agonist identified to date, being 50-fold more selective than salbutamol itself (Table 3).

Affinity and efficacy

The affinity of a ligand is a measure of the avidity of its binding to its receptor. Few β_2-agonists have been shown to have a much higher affinity than isoprenaline and, indeed, salbutamol, has a relatively low affinity for β_2-adrenoceptors. In contrast, salmeterol has high affinity for the β_2-adrenoceptor, with a Ki of 53 nM, compared with 200 and 2500 nM for isoprenaline and salbutamol, respectively [30].

Table 3. Comparative β-adrenoceptor pharmacology of salmeterol

	β_1-Adrenoceptors (Atria: inotropic activity)		β_2-Adrenoceptors (Bronchus: relaxant activity)		Selectivity
β-Agonist	Relative Potency	Efficacy	Relative Potency	Efficacy	$\beta_2 : \beta_1$
Isoprenaline	1.0	100	1.0	100	1.0
Salbutamol	0.0004	14	0.55	86	1375
Fenoterol	0.005	100	0.6	100	120
Formoterol	0.05	100	20.0	100	400
Salmeterol	0.0001	4	8.5	63	85,000

β-adrenoceptor potency, however, is a function, not only of receptor affinity, but also of receptor efficacy. A full agonist will have a high efficacy, while a pure antagonist will have low or zero efficacy. The majority of β_2-adrenoceptor agonists have an intermediate efficacy, and if tissue factors permit, they will behave as full agonists, but if receptor density is too low, or coupling is inadequate, the β-agonist may behave in a partial manner, i.e., it will be incapable of achieving the same maximum effect as an agonist of higher efficacy, and it may even behave as an antagonist. Examples of compounds of high efficacy (approximately equivalent to isoprenaline) are procaterol, fenoterol and formoterol (Table 3); whereas most saligenins and resorcinols, salbutamol and terbutaline, for example, tend to be of moderate efficacy (65–85 %), and the efficacy of the dichloroaniline, clenbuterol, is low (40 %). Salmeterol has an efficacy at β_2-adrenoceptors in airways smooth muscle of ca. 65 % [30]. Low efficacy in a β_2-adrenoceptor agonist does not, however, compromise its clinical effectiveness as a bronchodilator drug. The efficacy of β_2-agonists at extrapulmonary β-adrenoceptors, may, however, be of clinical importance. For example, fenoterol and formoterol have the same efficacy as isoprenaline at cardiac β_1-adrenoceptors (Table 3), whereas salbutamol is a partial agonist and salmeterol has very low efficacy (Table 3). Clinical studies have recently confirmed these differences between fenoterol, formoterol and salbutamol [31].

Onset and duration of action

In addition to differences in receptor affinity, efficacy and selectivity, the novel mechanism of action of salmeterol has resulted in a pharmacodynamic profile (rate of onset and duration of action) which is clearly different from other β_2-agonists. For example, in isolated airway preparations, containing β_2-adrènoceptors, such as the guinea pig trachea and human bronchial smooth muscle in vitro, the onset of action of isoprenaline, salbutamol, terbutaline and fenoterol is rapid (<4 min), that of formoterol is somewhat delayed (>5 min) and responses to salmeterol (Table 4) are slow to each equilibrium under these conditions (> 30 min). These differences are not so apparent clinically, however

Table 4

	Human Bronchus			Asthmatic Patients		
β_2-agonist	EC_{50} (nM)	Onset of action (min)	Duration of action (min)	Dose (μg)	Onset of action (min)*	Duration of action (hours)*
Salbutamol	200	3.3	6.8	200	5–7	4–6
Formoterol	2	5.3	6.6	24	6–8	10–12
Salmeterol	5	35.6	> 240	50	15–17	> 12

* FEV_1 > 15 % increase over baseline

(Table 4), where, for example, the time to 15 % increase in FEV_1 following a 50 μg dose of salmeterol in only a few minutes slower than with a standard 200 μg dose of salbutamol [33]. In contrast, there are marked differences in the duration of action of β_2-agonists. While isoprenaline has a short duration of action, and equipotent concentrations of salbutamol, fenoterol, and formoterol (Table 4) are similar (< 20 min), the relaxant effects of salmeterol on airways smooth muscle are long-lasting (>7 h). The duration of action of β_2-agonists against spasmogen-induced, neuronally mediated, and inherent tone in the human bronchus is in the order: salmeterol ≫ formoterol ≥ salbutamol ≥ terbutaline > fenoterol [30]. In contrast, in tissues containing predominantly β_1 or β_3-adrenoceptors, salmeterol is short-acting [17, 34], again supporting the concept that the mechanism of action (exosite binding) is specific to β_2-receptors. Indeed, salmeterol has the longest-acting relaxant effects on human airways smooth muscle of any β-agonist, but despite this long duration of action, there is no evidence of tachyphylaxis to its bronchodilator effects.

Analysis of the pharmacodynamic data, has revealed a further difference with salmeterol from other β_2-agonists. Whereas the duration of action of salbutamol and formoterol can be increased by increasing the concentration applied to the tissue, salmeterol appears to be inherently long-acting, in that its effects are independent of the concentration applied to the tissue [30]. These differences have been confirmed in asthmatic patients, where the onset and duration of action of formoterol are dependent on the dose administered (Fig. 3), whilst bronchodilation in response to salmeterol is independent of dose (Fig. 3).

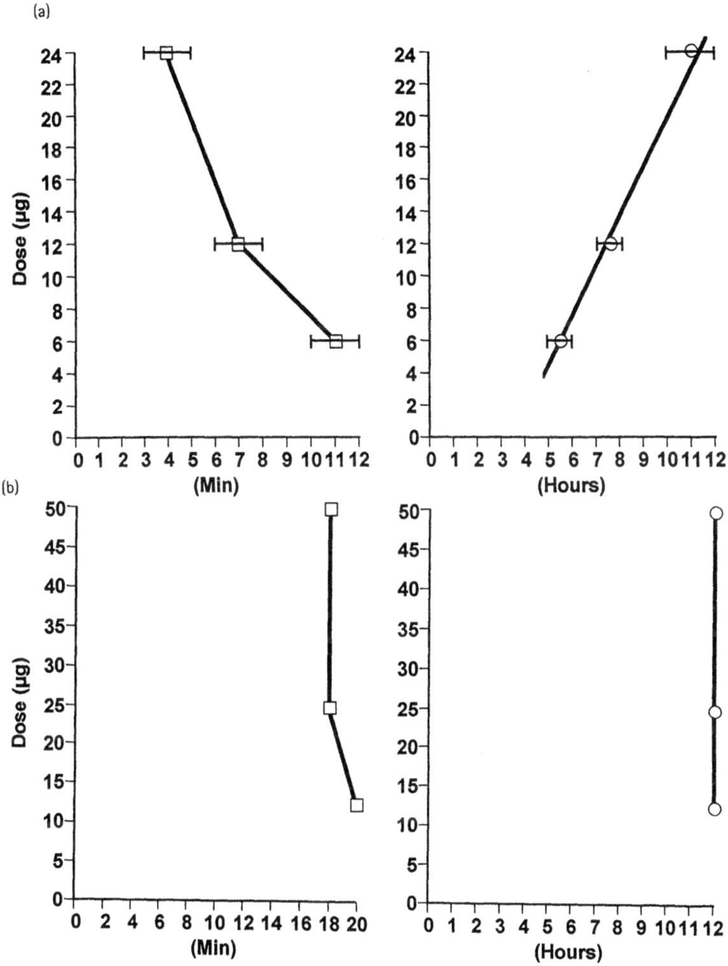

Fig. 3. (a) Dose-dependent decrease in onset and increase in duration of bronchodilatation in asthmatic patients in response to formoterol (6–24 μg); (b) Dose-independent onset and duration of bronchodilator responses to salmeterol (12.5–50 μg) in asthmatic patients

The pharmacodynamic profile of slower onset in action, and an inherently long duration of effect is consistent with the exo-site mechanism, of action of salmeterol. This profile also allows us to differentiate between β-agonists like salbutamol which are used for rapid relief of acute bronchospasm (Table 4), and salmeterol, which is aimed at twice-daily maintenance therapy, and where the slower onset of action is not a factor, and the key element is the long duration of effect (Table 4). However, in clinical practice, it is likely that, on occasions, both drugs will be used together – for example, in the asthmatic patient taking salmeterol who requires use of a short-acting β-agonist to control breakthrough symptoms. It is therefore important to demonstrate that in the presence of an ongoing response to salmeterol, there is a normal and full relaxation of human airway tissue to salbutamol. In such studies, the response to salbutamol was the same both before and after salmeterol [30]. This experimental finding has been confirmed in the extensive clinical trial programme on salmeterol [35]. Indeed, at the clinical dose of 50 μg, studies have shown salmeterol to occupy only 4 % of the total number of β_2-receptors in the lung, implying that there is a large unoccupied receptor reserve for salbutamol and other short-acting β_2-agonists to interact with.

Bronchodilator activity

In human airways smooth muscle, salmeterol is of similar potency to isoprenaline, while salbutamol is at least 10 times less potent [30]. The maximal degree of relaxation induced by salmeterol is consistently less than that of isoprenaline and salbutamol indicating the partial agonist nature of the response. Salbutamol, fenoterol and formoterol have short durations of action, whereas salmeterol has a duration of effect in excess of 7 h [30].

Bronchodilation

Nebulised aerosol administration of β-agonists causes dose-related protection against histamine-induced bronchoconstriction in animal models. At equivalent threshold effective doses, salbutamol, salmeterol and formoterol result in similar maximal degrees of bronchodilation. Salbutamol has a duration of action of less than 1.5 h, and even after administration of doses 10-fold greater, this is still less than 3 h under these conditions [36]. Formoterol is longer-acting than salbutamol, its activity again appearing to be dose-related. In contrast, as predicted

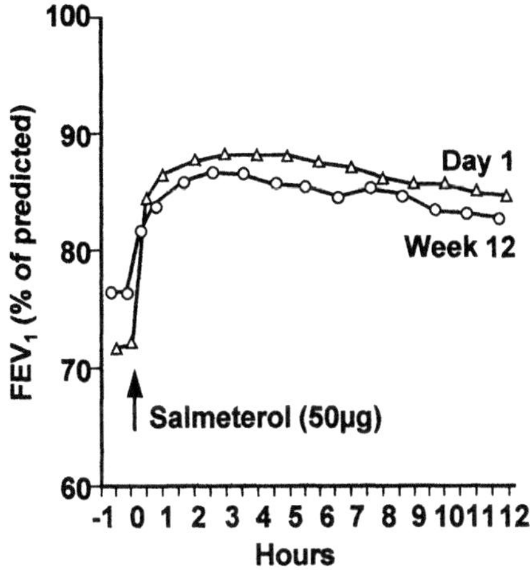

Fig. 4. Sustained bronchodilator responses to salmeterol in asthmatic patients when administered 50 μg b. d for 12 weeks

from its in vitro activity on isolated airways smooth muscle, the bronchodilator effects of salmeterol are apparent for at least 6 h at all dose levels [36]. These differences between the profile of action of salmeterol and other β_2-agonists have been extrapolated to man and to the asthmatic patient in a number of extensive clinical trials (Fig. 4).

Non-bronchodilator properties

The pharmacological activity of β_2-agonists is not restricted to airways smooth muscle and they also exhibit a range of non-bronchodilator properties. For example, there is experimental evidence that β-agonists can inhibit acute inflammatory responses in the lung, subcutaneous tissues, and the skin following local, topical or oral administration; data arising from studies both in animals and in man [37]. Clinical evidence, however, has not shown currently available β_2-agonists to have significant anti-inflammatory activity in the lung. Recent evidence from preclinical and clinical studies [38], suggests that the lack of anti-inflammatory activity of first generation β_2-agonists may be a consequence of their short duration of action, since even the processes involved in acute inflammation can be slow to develop and resolve.

The second generation of β_2-adrenoceptor agonists, represented by salmeterol, are both more potent, and more importantly, longer-acting than the first generation compounds such as salbutamol and terbutaline, and appear to exhibit more significant non-bronchodilator activity.

Mast cells and inflammatory mediator release

Salmeterol is potent in inhibiting antigen-induced histamine, leukotriene C_4 and D_4 and prostaglandin D_2 release from human lung tissue in vitro, with a 50 % inhibitory concentration range of 1–3 nM [39]. The rank order of potency is: formoterol > salmeterol ≥ isoprenaline > salbutamol, but all the drugs are capable of producing complete inhibition of mediator release. As in airway preparations, and in marked contrast to short-acting β_2-agonists which are active for only up to 4 h, salmeterol has a sustained effect, suppressing inflammatory mediator release for > 20 h, while the duration of action of formoterol (8 h) is intermediate between that of salmeterol and salbutamol [39].

Endothelial cells: Vascular permeability

Salmeterol exhibits a concentration-dependent inhibition of thrombin-stimulated albumin transport through endothelial cell monolayers in culture with an EC_{50} of 2.6 nM, compared with 100 nM for isoprenaline [40].

At bronchodilator doses by the inhaled route, salmeterol inhibits vascular permeability in the lung in vivo and similar findings have been reported for salbutamol and formoterol [41]. Similarly, in the skin, inhibition of histamine and bradykinin-induced vascular permeability by intradermal administration of salbutamol, salmeterol or formoterol has been reported [42]. Again, differences in duration of action for the effect of β_2-agonists on vascular permeability in both the lung and skin were observed, in the rank order salmeterol > formoterol > salbutamol with the effects of salmeterol being apparent for up to 8 h [41].

Inflammatory cells

In experimental studies, the property of long-acting β_2-agonists, such as salmeterol, which most distinguishes them from the first generation short-acting drugs is their ability to inhibit the accumulation of granulocytes at sites of acute inflammation. Local administration of low concentrations of salmeterol (10 nM) inhibits both plasma exudation and leukocyte emigration induced by inflammatory stimuli in the intact microcirculation [43]. At bronchodilator doses in the guinea pig in vivo, salmeterol inhibits both neutrophil accumulation in the airways in response to lipopolysaccharide [44], and attenuates eosinophil infiltration into the lung, which occurs 24 h following challenge with platelet activating factor or antigen, while salbutamol is without effect [45].

The inhibitory effects of salmeterol on cell accumulation is unlikely to be due to a direct action on inflammatory cells, since they are relatively insensitive to inhibition with this type of drug, requiring the use of high concentrations (> 10^{-6}M). Although inhibitory effects have been reported against LTB_4 synthesis in neutrophils [46], ECP release from eosinophils [47], TxB_2 formation by alveolar macrophages [48] and anti-CD_3-induced lymphocyte proliferation [49], these effects are only modest. Instead an effect on the vascular endothelium, in addition to attenuating plasma protein extravasation, may also explain the observed actions of salmeterol on granulocyte accumulation, since inflammatory cells diapedese into tissues through the same tight junctions between endothelial cells, and the inhibition of these two acute inflammatory processes may therefore be through a common mechanism. Indeed, β_2-agonists, like salbutamol and salmeterol, increase intracellular cyclic AMP in endothelial cells in culture [50]. The rank order of potency is: salmeterol > isoprenaline > salbutamol. By increasing intracellular cyclic AMP, it is possible that salmeterol may act as a functional antagonist to prevent the shape change induced by inflammatory stimuli, thereby maintaining the integrity of the endothelium and inhibiting the recruitment of eosinophils and neutrophils.

Bronchial epithelium

The bronchial epithelium also contains functional β-adrenoceptors and long-acting β_2-agonists, like salmeterol, may therefore also be effective in modulating some of the consequences of acute inflammation at the level of epithelial cell.

Until recently, little attention has been paid to the effects of β_2-adrenoceptors agonists on cilial function. However, salbutamol and salmeterol have now both been shown to increase cilial beat frequency (CBF) in human nasal and bronchial epithelial cells in culture, with salmeterol being more potent than salbutamol [51]. The effects of salbutamol are modest and transient (< 2 h) in nature, whereas salmeterol produced an increment in CBF in bronchial epithelium from 9.2 to 10.9 Hz, at 100-fold lower concentration, and its effect was sustained for 15–20 h. Salmeterol exhibits a concentration-dependent inhibition of the ciliary dyskinesia induced by prolonged contact with the ciliotoxins, pyocyanin or rhamnolipid [52]. In addition, a protective effective of salmeterol against the cellular damage induced by micro-organisms such as *Pseudomonas aeruginosa* and *Haemophilus influenzae* has also been reported [53].

Experimentally, therefore, in addition to its long-lasting effects on airways smooth muscle, salmeterol, by acting as a functional antagonist, can be shown to inhibit a number of processes involved in acute inflammation, a profile which was not predicted at the outset of the research programme in 1980. Its sustained effects on mediator release, cell recruitment and vascular permeability are more apparent than those of drugs with reported anti-inflammatory activity such as ketotifen, theophylline, and sodium cromoglycate and may have important implications for the use of salmeterol in prophylactic therapy. However, the profile of activity of salmeterol is likely to be different from that of corticosteroids, which are more effective against chronic inflammation. Salmeterol should be seen, therefore, not as a replacement, but rather as potentially complementary to steroids.

Clinical experience with salmeterol

The long-acting β_2-adrenoceptor agonists were developed specifically for inhaled use as twice daily maintenance therapy in the treatment of reversible airways obstruction. Clinical studies for up to 5 years duration, in many thousands of patients, have confirmed the pharmacological predictions made for salmeterol. It is highly efficacious in bronchial asthma, producing sustained bronchodilation after aerosol administration [54]. The onset of bronchodilation is slower (by 3–10 min) with salmeterol (50 μg) than with salbutamol (200 μg), although this may be of little clinical importance, as salmeterol is intended for maintenance therapy and not as symptomatic relief. Peak bronchodilation at 1 h is of similar magnitude to salbutamol, but the duration of action of salmeterol is much longer, FEV_1 remaining > 15 % over baseline values for 14 h, compared with 4–6 h for salbutamol (Fig. 3). Salmeterol, at 50 and 100 μg doses, protected against methacholine or histamine challenge for > 12 h [55]. Similarly, in a study in which exercise challenge was employed, whereas salbutamol was effective at 1 h, but not at 6 and 12 h, salmeterol was active for at least 12 h [56]. This was also observed in paediatric studies. Multicenter European dose-ranging studies using 12.5–200 μg, have shown that salmeterol, 50 μg twice daily, is the optimum therapeutic dosage in the treatment of mild to moderate asthma, reducing diurnal variation and leading to a progressive improvement in lung function, with 100 μg twice daily providing further benefit in patients with more severe disease [57]. There was no indication of tachyphylaxis to the pulmonary effects of salmeterol following administration for up to 12 weeks and longer (Fig. 4). Similarly, no evidence of rebound deterioration of lung function was observed after withdrawal of salmeterol treatment.

One of the objectives in developing long-acting β_2-agonists was to be able to control the symptoms of nocturnal asthma. In patients, who were experiencing approximately 80 % weekly awakenings due to asthma, both 50 and 100 μg of salmeterol had a significant effect, with the higher dose eliminating the symptoms of nocturnal asthma within 7 days of starting treatment [58].

Recent analysis of long-term studies (> 12 months) has revealed that asthma exacerbations are less in salmeterol-treated patients, and remain low whether or not inhaled corticosteroids were taken concurrently [59]. There is also evidence that salmeterol improves the quality of life in asthmatic patients, compared with their existing therapy [60].

Conclusions

The objective of developing a drug with therapeutically significant, sustained bronchodilator activity for the treatment of reversible airways obstruction, when administered by the inhaled route, has been achieved in the new generation of long-acting β_2-agonists, represented by salmeterol. As a result of potent and prolonged activation of β_2-adrenoceptors in airways smooth muscle, salmeterol produces bronchodilation for at least 12 h. This pharmacological activity arises from the novel mechanism of action of salmeterol, whereby as a direct consequence of the design features of the molecule, it is localised in a specific exo-site domain of the β_2-receptor protein, from where it can continuously stimulate the active site of the receptor.

References

1. Holgate ST (1988) Postgrad Med J 64: 82
2. Gay LN, Long JW (1949) J Am Med Assoc 139: 452
3. Lands AM, Arnold A, McAuliff JP, Luduena FP, Brown TG (1967) Nature 214: 597
4. Brittain RT, Jack D, Richie AC (1970) Adv Drug Res 5: 197
5. Sustained release salbutamol was marketed as Volmax™
6. Friedel HA, Brogden RN (1988) Drugs 35: 22
7. Pedersen BK, Laursen LC, Gnosspelius Y, Faurschou P, Weeke B (1985) Eur J Clin Pharm 29: 25
8. Brittain RT (1990) Lung 168: 111
9. Lal S, Dash CH, Gribben MD (1974) Thorax 29: 317
10. Wallis CJ (1993) Actual Chim Thér 20: 265
11. Rhodes DG, Newton RF, Butler R, Herbette L (1993) Mol Pharm 42: 596
12. Herbette LG, Trumborne M, Chester DW, Katz AM (1988) Mol Cell Cardiol 20: 373
13. Stadel JM, Nakeda MT (1991) β-adrenoceptors: Mol Biol Biochem Pharmacol 7: 26
14. Tota MR, Candelore MR, Dixon RAF, Strader CD (1991) Trends Pharmacol Sci 12: 4
15. Strader CD, Candelore MR, Hill WS, Sigal IS, Dixon RAF (1989) J Biol Chem 264: 13572
16. Lewell XQ (1992) Drug Design & Discovery 9: 29
17. Swales N, Patterson G (1990) Br J Pharmacol 100: 489 P
18. Nials AT, Sumner MJ, Johnson M, Coleman RA (1993) Br J Pharmacol 108: 507

19. Bradshaw J, Brittain RT, Coleman RA et al (1987) Br J Pharmacol 92: 590 P
20. Johnson M (1992) In: New drugs for asthma, IBC Technical Services, London, p 18
21. Nials AT, Barker RC, Coleman RA, Vardey CJ (1994) Am J Resp Crit Care Med A 482
22. Johnson M (1992) In: Costello JF, Mann RD (eds) β-adrenoceptor agonists in the treatment of asthma. Parthenon, U. K., p 27
23. Anderson GP (1993) Life Sci 52: 2145
24. Jack D (1991) Br J Clin Pharmacol 31: 501
25. Green SA, Spasoff AP, Coleman RA, Johnson M, Liggett SB (1996) J Biol Chem 271: 24029
26. Coleman RA, Johnson M, Nials AT, Vardey CJ (1996) Trends Pharmacol Sci 17: 324
27. Johnson M (1991) Agents and Actions 34: 79
28. Lipworth BJ (1992) Drug Safety 7: 54
29. Reeds PJ, Hay SM, Dorward PM, Palmer RM (1988) Comp Biochem Physiol 89: 337
30. Johnson M, Butchers PR, Coleman RA et al (1993) Life Sciences 26: 2131
31. Bremner P, Woodman K, Burgess C et al (1993) Eur Resp J 6: 204
32. Johnson M (1991) Eur Resp Rev 1: 253
33. Palmer JBD (1991) In: Salmeterol: a reappraisal of asthma management. Medicine Group, Oxford, 1991, p 5
34. Patel V, Martin DP, Coates J, Strong P (1992) Br J Pharmacol 106: 275
35. Palmer JBD (1991) Eur Resp Rev 1: 297
36. Ball DI, Brittain RT, Coleman RA et al (1991) Br J Pharmacol 104: 665
37. Archer CB, MacDonald DM (1987) Clin Exp Dermatol 12: 323
38. Johnson M, Vardey CJ, Whelan CJ (1992) Clin Exp Allergy 22: 177
39. Butchers PR, Vardey CJ, Johnson M (1991) Br J Pharmacol 104: 672
40. Allen MJ, Vardey CJ, Coleman RA (1994) Am J Resp Crit Care Med 149: A 819
41. Whelan CJ, Johnson M (1992) Br J Pharmacol 105: 831
42. Chung KF, Barnes PJ (1991) In: Agents & Actions 34: 97
43. Dahlen SE, Raud J, Palmertz U, Hedquist P (1991) Am Rev Resp Dis 145: A 741
44. Whelan CJ, Johnson M, Vardey CJ (1993) Am Rev Resp Dis 147: A 62
45. Whelan CJ, Johnson M (1991) Eur Resp J 4: 166 S
46. Johnson M (1990) Lung 168: 115
47. Rabe K (1990) Am Rev Resp Dis 141: A 29
48. Baker AJ, Fuller RW (1990) Am Rev Resp Dis 141: A 394
49. Oddera S, Silvestri M, Lantero S, Queglia R, Testi R, Rossi GA (1994) Am J Resp Crit Care Med 149: A 805
50. McCrea KE, Hill SJ (1993) Br J Pharmacol 110: 619

51. Rusnak C, Sapsford RJ, Devalia JL, Davies RJ (1990) Am Rev Resp Dis 141: A 1030
52. Kanthakumar K, Cundell DR, Johnson M, Willis PJ, Taylor GW, McCole PJ, Wilson R (1993) Br J Pharmacol 112: 493
53. Dowling RB, Rayner CFJ, Rutman A, Jackson AD, Kanthakumar K, Dewar A, Taylor GW, Cole PJ, Johnson M, Wilson R (1997) Am J Resp Crit Care Med 155: 327
54. Britton M (1991) Eur Resp Rev 1: 288
55. Pauwels R (1991) In: Salmeterol; a reappraisal of asthma management. The Medicine Group, Oxford, p 9
56. Dhillon DP (1991) Eur Resp Rev 1: 265
57. Brogden RN, Faulds D (1991) Drugs 42: 895
58. Douglas NJ, Fitzpatrick MF (1992) Eur Resp Rev 1: 293
59. Fuller RW (1991) In: Salmeterol: a reappraisal of asthma management. The Medicine Group, Oxford, p 18
60. Palmer JBD, Hyland ME (1992) Eur Resp Rev 1: 301

Correspondence: Dr. Malcolm Johnson, Glaxo Wellcome Research & Development, Stockley Park West, Uxbridge, Middlesex UB11 1BT, U.K.

Discussion

Dr. Block: Thank you, Malcolm! Dr. Anderson, may I ask you the first question: You mentioned the method of freeze-fractioning of biomembranes in response to the compound that you are studying. Is there a certain correlation between the changes that you observed in the presence of the beta adrenergic compound that you studied and the surface charges being measured?

Dr. Anderson: The technique is not freeze-fraction. These are living cells and we used an argon laser to excite the cells at 630 nanometers. The technique uses a molecule which changes the clarity of light which shines through the cells. When a second drug is introduced, the angle of clarity changes, which allows you to measure the association of the second drug to the membrane. So all of those cells were living. In that biophysical table were very complex data, but if anyone who has a bend for biophysics, he would have noticed that the mechanisms of action of formoterol and salmeterol are very very different. We believe that salmeterol behaves somewhat like hexane, it has a natural affinity to lipid, whereas formoterol does not have the same biophysics at all. And what we believe happens is that it actually complexes water molecules around it and when it approaches the lipid membrane the water is freed, releasing energy, so the molecule moves into the cell. But that's why the interaction is unstable and reversible.

Dr. Block: If you look at the efficacy of your compound as compared to the different physical chemical changes and biophysical changes, are there effects of both compounds related to the transport change of sodium or potassium?

Dr. Anderson: I think there are differences. Cook's work shows that there is no change in the potassium conductance with salmeterol at all. There is no activation in BK channels (BKC), Formoterol probably does activate, but I think it's good evidence against the BKC hypothesis, actually, because salmeterol is so effective in the clinic that BK channels could not be relevant to human conditions.

Dr. Block: Would you like to comment, Dr. Johnson?

Dr. Johnson: Just about what Gary has just said. I think that where people have studied BK channel opening with beta agonists, it probably plays a very trivial role in their bronchodilator activity. But if it occurs at all, it occurs with a higher efficacy agonist. They didn't study formoterol, but they studied isoprenaline and this did have some opening effect on the channel. Salbutamol was less effective and salmeterol, a good bronchodilator, does not open the BK channel at all.

Dr. Block: Let me just ask one more question. The final experiment that you mentioned was a very interesting one, because you know we both have a certain interest in finding the mechanism of cell protection, especially in those circumstances. Has someone looked at the ability of haemophilus to affect adhesion molecules in the presence of beta adrenergic agonists?

Dr. Johnson: Not specifically, but again, very interestingly, what they did in these experiments was to actually count the number of microorganisms that were adhering to the mucosa. And that was not affected at all by the presence of salmeterol.

Dr. Block: It was not?

Dr. Johnson: It was not. So salmeterol doesn't inhibit the binding or the adhesion of the micro-organism. But what it does in some way is to influence the events which occur subsequent to that interaction. Robert Wilson has studied this phenomenon. When the micro-organism is damaging the mucosa, cyclic AMP levels fall in the cell. What this drug is probably doing is that it is maintaining those levels to a point where there is some sort of cyto-protection.

But the most intriguing thing is that these experiments have been repeated putting neutrophil elastase onto the mucosa. Elastase causes significant damage on its own, but that again is completely inhibited in the presence of salmeterol. So this is a cytoprotective effect against protease enzymes as well as against micro-organisms. He hasn't looked at formoterol but I suspect he'd see the same thing. I think it's intriguing that the more you study these long-acting ß-2-agonist molecules, they are more than bronchodilators. No-one is necessarily claiming anti-inflammatory activity, but there are other consequences for raising cyclic AMP.

Dr. Greening: I was hoping that Dr. Anderson could have told me a little bit more about formoterol, because following on from Ian Adcock's presentation, and seeing the full agonist effect of formoterol, and indeed, some beta-1 similarities with formoterol and isoprenaline, I wondered what information you could tell us with formoterol in terms of stimulation of CREB, and interaction with glucocorticoids.

Dr. Anderson: We have no data on what formoterol does to CREB at all. So we don't know. We do know in the clinic that formoterol doesn't cause any exacerbations of disease whatsoever. And it doesn't have a negative interaction with corticosteroids. So we do know that.

Dr. Greening: I'm glad my patients don't have PhD's in pharmacology, because they'd get very confused about things, but they know that drugs work.

Dr. Götz: Can I just come back to the last slide of Dr. Johnson's, which I think is for a clinician very exciting. Have you comparative data of salmeterol with salbutamol, and what is the effect of them on muco-ciliary clearance? Obviously you would assume that salmeterol is going to stimulate clearance, so as to eradicate part of the infection there. Do you have any data there?

Dr. Johnson: Well, again, this is all data from Robert Wilson's laboratory. He has compared salmeterol with salbutamol and in fact salbutamol has a very weak effect in protecting cells against the micro-organisms. That's probably no surprise because this damage occurs over a 6- to 10-hour period, and you require the drug to be able to raise cyclic AMP for that period of time.

What two groups have previously shown is that salmeterol does stimulate cilial activity by increasing cilial beat frequency. We are doing some studies now with Michael Newhouse in Canada, looking at muco-ciliary transport in man with salmeterol because the first study was done under organ culture conditions. It may be possible that in the patient, clearance of the micro-organisms may actually add to this picture.

Dr. Block: Maybe a very short question before we go on. You mentioned a certain amount, I think about 4% of beta-adrenergic sites are being occupied in the presence of salmeterol. As far as my recollection goes, under physiological conditions, receptors generally are expressed at a very low level, even lesser than 4 per cent, because as I know especially dealing with cholesterol transport, they are less than one per cent expressed even under maximum stimulatory conditions.

Dr. Johnson: No, this wasn't measuring the level of expression of the receptors. This was looking at the occupancy or calculating the occupancy. Obviously it's very difficult to actually measure occupancy in the patient. Using PET scanning, they had estimated the density of beta-2 receptors in the patient's lung and from the concentration of salmeterol, the receptor occupancy could be calculated.

The difficulty with the PET data is that it gives total lung receptors. It doesn't have the resolution to look in the airway. But my thesis would be that even if the occupancy was ten times higher, if it was 40 per cent, there would still be 60 per cent receptors left for salbutamol. I think that explains the clinical data, that patients on salmeterol respond quite normally to a short-acting beta-agonist.

Development of bambuterol; a long acting, orally active beta-agonist prodrug

L.-Å. Svensson

Department of Medicinal Chemistry,
Astra Draco AB, Lund, Sweden

Summary

Bambuterol, Bambec®, is a novel, orally active, long-acting bronchodilator with 24 hours duration of action and a lower incidence of adverse advents as compared with other oral bronchodilators [1]. Bambuterol, dimethylcarbamic acid 5-[2-[(1,1-dimethylethyl)amino]-1-hydroxyethyl]-1,3-phenylene ester, is a prodrug to the β_2-adrenoceptor agonist terbutaline. It was developed by Astra Draco AB, and is currently approved for the treatment of bronchial asthma, chronic bronchitis and other lung diseases, where bronchospasm is a complicating factor.

This paper reviews how bambuterol was developed from terbutaline by use of the prodrug technique.

The prodrug approach

The term prodrug is used to describe an agent which must undergo chemical or enzymatic transformation from a biologically inactive compound to the active drug after administration, so that the metabolic product, or active drug, can subsequently exhibit the desired pharmacological response.

This technique could be used to temporarily alter and so optimize the physicochemical properties and, thus, the pharmacological and toxicological profiles of an agent.
Thus, when the active drug is not fully utilized because of some identifiable barrier or problem, the physicochemical properties of the drug can be altered by attachment of a pro-moiety. This allows the prodrug to bypass the barrier, and once past the barrier, to revert to the active drug, or parent compound, by a postbarrier enzyme or nonenzymatic process. The prodrug technique could also be used to facilitate transport of the pharmacologically inactive prodrug to its target tissue where it then is converted to active drug.

The prodrug technique requires a parent compound with adequate pharmacological properties and suitable molecular structure, so that chemical manipulations can be performed to improve pharmacokinetic properties.

Terbutaline (Bricanyl®) (Fig. 1), which was developed in our laboratories 25 years ago, fulfilled the requirements of a parent drug. It is a clinically well documented selective β_2-agonist bronchodilator and, being a resorcinol derivative, it has two phenolic hydroxyl groups which are suitable for prodrug manipulations.

Since prodrugs usually are inactive *per se* and need bioactivation to generate the pharmacologically active compound, one has to consider this fact when choosing the kind of chemistry to be involved in the bioactivation process. The type of prodrug derivative we decided to work with was of the ester type since phenolic esters are known to be substrates for esterases in the human body. Esterases are widespread in the human organism and they are very efficient in hydrolyzing various esters.

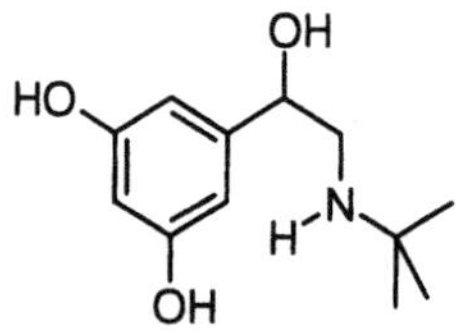

Fig. 1. Terbutaline

Rate control of esterase catalyzed ester hydrolysis

As a first step, a series of simple fatty acid ester prodrugs of terbutaline were prepared in order to examine to what extent it was possible to control the rate of the esterase catalyzed hydrolysis. With the aim to improve absorption and bioavailability of terbutaline, we also were interested in finding out if such prodrugs could be used to diminish first-pass conjugation of terbutaline.

As can be seen from Table 1, it is possible to control the rate of esterase catalyzed hydrolysis of such esters, but their half-life in human blood *in vitro* is only a few minutes [2].

In man, both improved absorption as well as increased bioavailability was achieved with one of these ester prodrugs; ibuterol [3]. These improvements however did not offer any therapeutic advantages, since systemic side effects, such as tremor, became disturbing when the plasma concentration of terbutaline peaked, and the duration of action surprisingly was shorter than when terbutaline was administered as such.

In spite of these disappointing results, an important observation was made with this prodrug; the rather weak lung-uptake of terbutaline

Table 1. Rates of hydrolysis of a series of terbutaline ester prodrugs in human plasma

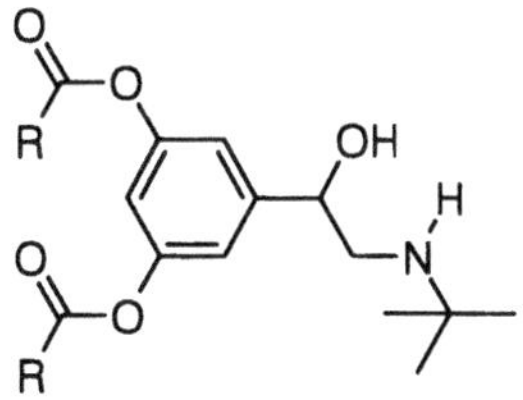

R	V_m/K_m ($s^{-1}10^3$)
CH_3–	10.0
CH_3CH_2–	14.0
$(CH_3)_2CH$- (ibuterol)	4.4
$CH_3CH_2(CH_3)CH$-	0.6
$(CH_3)_3C$-	0.04

increased dramatically when it was converted into its bis-isobutyrate prodrug; ibuterol. In the isolated, perfused guinea-pig and rat lungs, lung extraction of terbutaline was only 0.013+/–0.003 (rat) and 0.021+/–0.005 (guinea-pig), while ibuterol displayed a considerably higher lung uptake; 0.41+/–0.01 (rat) and 0.36+/–0.01 (guinea-pig) [4].

Thus, it is obvious that by increasing the lipophilicity of terbutaline, the lung extraction increases. It was also found that ibuterol was rapidly converted to terbutaline in lung tissue.

The problem with ibuterol and related prodrugs of terbutaline, is that they are too rapidly hydrolyzed by esterases in the gut wall, in the liver and in the blood. Therefore, the systemic availability of these ester prodrugs were negligible after oral administration, and the unique lung distribution properties of the prodrug could not be taken advantage of.

Thus, ester prodrugs with increased hydrolytic stability had to be sought for.

Increased hydrolytic stability *in vitro* in human plasma could be obtained with the benzoic acid ester derivatives [5] (Fig. 2).

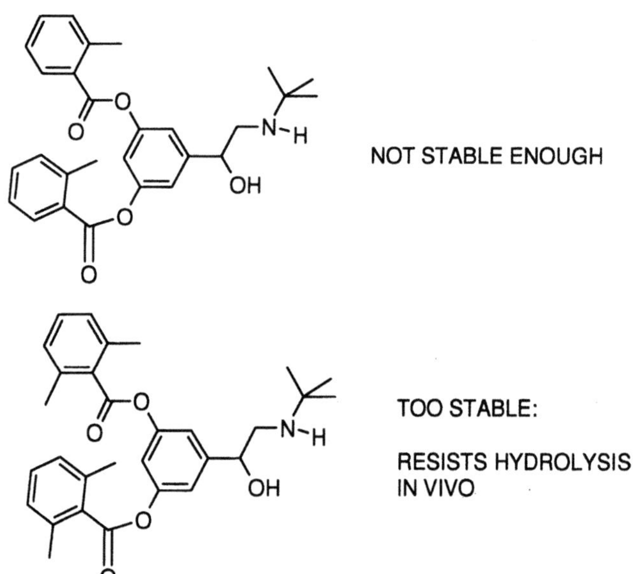

Fig. 2. Terbutaline benzoate prodrugs

The half-lives for formation of terbutaline from such ester prodrugs in human plasma were of the order 1 to 2 h. However, by increasing the steric hindrance near the ester carbonyl group by 2,6-dimethyl substitution, an ester prodrug of extreme hydrolytic stability was obtained so that bioconversion to terbutaline *in vivo,* even in man, was hindered. On the other hand, the corresponding 2-methyl-substituted derivatives probably did not have sufficient presystemic stability since it did not show sustained action in the dog, which is known to hydrolyze this type of ester at a rate about five times slower than man.

The cascade ester prodrug approach

Another attempt to design an ester prodrug with high presystemic stability was the cascade ester D2438 [5] (Fig. 3).

This prodrug was designed to undergo first-pass hydrolysis and conjugation at a site in the prodrug molecule distal from the active resorcinol moiety in terbutaline. The cascade ester is constructed from p-hydroxybenzoic acid and pivalic acid. Since the half-life of terbutaline bis-pivalate in human plasma is less than 5 min, but that of the bis-p-hydroxybenzoate is approximately 1 h, it is primarily the pivalate bond in the cascade ester that should undergo first-pass hydrolysis. We thus expected the cascade ester to undergo first-pass hydrolysis mainly at the p-pivaloyloxy bond, possibly followed by conjugation at the resulting

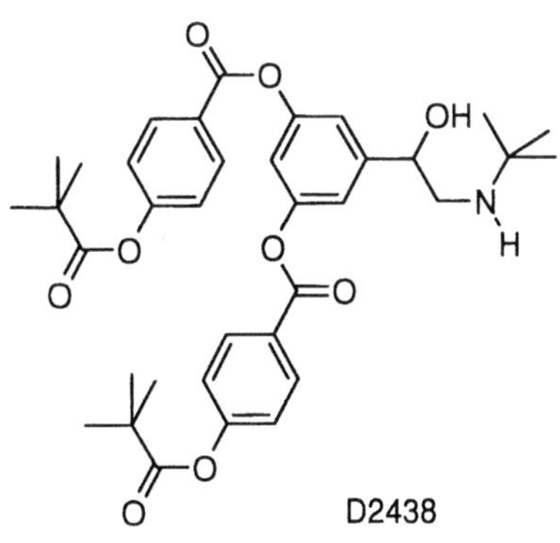

D2438

Fig. 3. The cascade ester approach

p-hydroxybenzoyl moiety. In this way the active resorcinol moiety in terbutaline should be protected during first pass, and eventually free terbutaline would be generated from free and conjugated p-hydroxybenzoates during and after the distribution phase.

The cascade ester turned out to be very stable in vitro in human plasma where a half-life of approximately 10 h was observed. Compared with a half-life of only a few seconds for ibuterol, the high stability displayed by D2438 was of an order that could be expected to protect the prodrug from extensive first-pass hydrolysis.

When D2438 was given orally to the dog we observed both sustained action and prolonged terbutaline plasma concentration profiles [6]. But, the hydrolysis of esters like these occurs slower in the dog than in man, and, in fact, disappointing results were obtained in man with oral D2438; neither sustained action nor prolonged terbutaline plasma concentration profiles were obtained.

Obviously, more sophisticated approaches than those previously used would have to be utilized to design ester prodrugs of terbutaline with adequate presystemic hydrolytic stability. The main problem clearly was how to achieve adequate ester bond stability so that the prodrug would resist hydrolysis by efficient esterases present in the gut wall and the liver.

The bambuterol approach

The high efficiency of the esterases to hydrolyze ester prodrugs eventually was overcome by the approach to build an esterase-inhibiting function into the prodrug molecule [6, 7]. In this way the prodrug could slow its own hydrolysis by inhibiting the esterases that attack it.

There is, however, one obstacle with this approach. A prodrug having a built-in esterase inhibiting function must exhibit a very high selectivity for the unspecific plasma cholinesterase. If acetylcholinesterase also is inhibited, increased levels of acetylcholine would result in a potentiation of asthmatic symptoms and, subsequently, in severe toxicity and CNS effects.

The selected compound, bambuterol (Fig. 4);
the *bis*-N,N-dimethylcarbamate of terbutaline, indeed was found to be

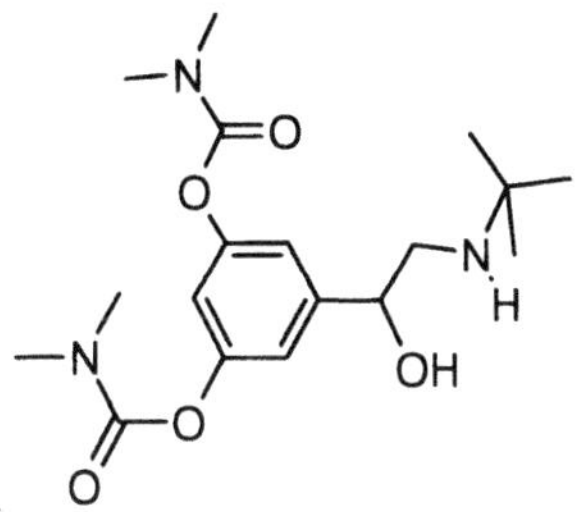

Fig. 4. Bambuterol

a very selective and potent inhibitor of human plasma cholinesterase with an IC50 value of 17 nM, while the corresponding value for acetyl cholinesterase was 2400-fold higher, i.e. 41 µM [8] . Bambuterol is also a safe inhibitor in man, since no effects were found that can be related to inhibition of acetyl cholinesterase [9].

Both terbutaline and bambuterol are used as racemates. (–)-Terbutaline is the enantiomer solely responsible for the pharmacological effect since it is more than 3000-fold as active as its (+)-enantiomer [10, 11]. Since (–)-terbutaline is formed from (–)-bambuterol, one could argue that bambuterol should be given as its pure (–)-enantiomer. However, both enantiomers may be needed for effective esterase inhibition, and also the (+)-enantiomer is a potent esterase inhibitor. The two bambuterol enantiomers thus display a slight but significant stereoselectivity in their interaction (hydrolysis and inhibition) with plasma cholinesterase; the IC50 is 2 nM for (–)-bambuterol, while it is 12–14 nM for (+)-bambuterol [12]. This difference in hydrolysis leads in fact to an increased formation of (–)-terbutaline from racemic bambuterol; the (–)/(+)-terbutaline ratio is 2.8 after bambuterol, while it is only about 2 after racemic terbutaline[12].

Hydrolysis turned out not to be the only bioactivating pathway for bambuterol. Human liver microsomal preparations have been demonstrated to partly hydrolyze bambuterol but also to catalyze an oxidative reaction at the carbamate methyl groups (Fig. 5).

In this way, by a combination of hydrolytic and oxidative metabolism, new carbamate metabolites are formed that are still prodrugs of

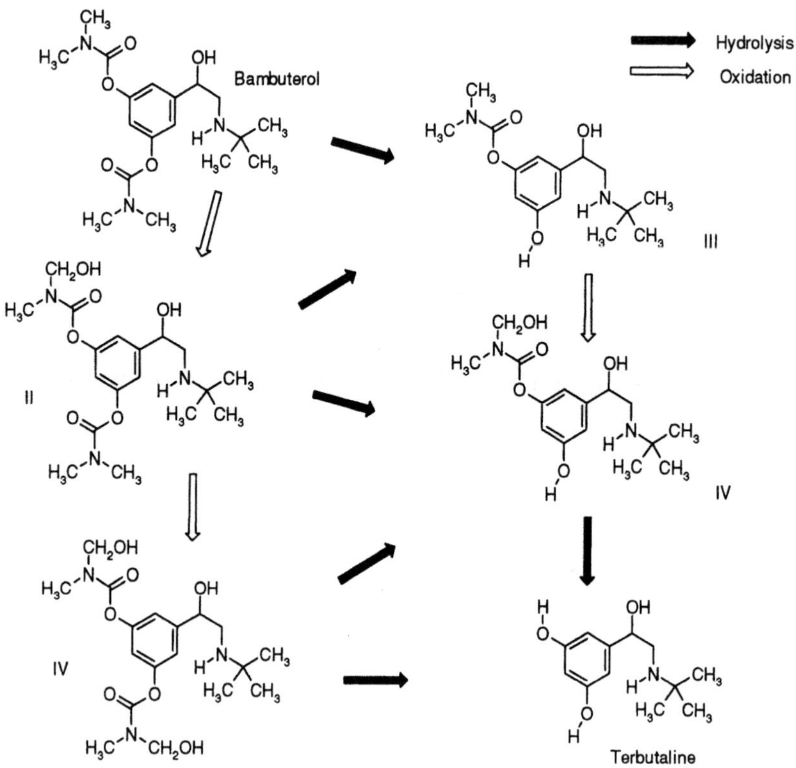

Fig. 5. Metabolic pathways of bambuterol

terbutaline and, hence, bambuterol is in fact a prodrug-prodrug[13, 14, 15]. The oxidation reaction is most likely catalyzed by the cytochrome P-450 dependent mixed function oxidases.

Interestingly, oxidation of the terbutaline part of bambuterol is no primary metabolic pathway.

Since two different metabolic pathways are involved in the bioconversion of bambuterol to terbutaline, variations in the activity of the two systems involved could lead to variations in the amount of terbutaline formed. However, a pharmacokinetic study in man revealed that although there was a large variation in the steady-state levels of metabolite III, (representing the hydrolytic pathway), and metabolite V, (representing the oxidative pathway), there was only a rather small variation in the level of terbutaline generated by bambuterol [16].

Patients having an impaired plasma cholinesterase activity, such as the atypical genotype, also produce the same amount of terbutaline as normal individuals [17], in spite of the fact that plasma from atypical subjects hydrolyses bambuterol slower than plasma from normal individuals [18]. The oxidative pathway may be an important metabolic route when cholinesterase activity is impaired.

Lung uptake mechanisms

Is there a specific uptake system in the lung for certain molecules? If so, what are the structural and physicochemical properties that are required to make use of this uptake system?

Several mechanisms seem to contribute to the lung uptake of weakly basic drugs, and some of these are commented on below.

Binding to phosphatidylserine

Yata and co-workers have studied phosphatidylserine as a determinant for the tissue distribution of weakly basic drugs in rats [19]. They estimated the *in vivo* tissue-to-plasma partition coefficient (K_P) values for quinidine, propranolol and imipramine, and when K_P was plotted against the concentration of phosphatidylserine in various tissues, a linear correlation was obtained. In another study from the same group [20], it was found that the phosphatidylserine concentration in alveolar macrophages was 10 times higher than in lung parenchyma. Again, the quinidine concentration was proportional to the concentration of phosphatidylserine vesicles. Furthermore, binding of weakly basic amines to phosphatidylserine seems to be stereoselective.

Binding to mitochondrial monoamineoxidase (MAO)

Hori and co-workers have reported that in an isolated lung perfusion method, basic drugs, such as imipramine, quinidine and metoclopramide, containing a cationic group and a lipophilic component, are selectively accumulated in the rat lung mitochondrial fraction [21, 22]. They were able to demonstrate that mitochondrial MAO has specific binding sites for basic drugs and hence may serve as a drug reservoir.

Chlorphentermine lung uptake

Chronic administration of chlorphentermine results in lung concentrations more than 100-times the concentration in plasma [23]. The accumulated drug exhibits widespread localization in the pulmonary tissue.

Active uptake mechanisms

Diamine and polyamines, such as putrescine and spermidine, are accumulated in the lung by a process that is energy-dependent and obeys saturation kinetic [24]. The reason why the herbicide and pulmonary toxicant paraquat is accumulated by the lung is that it is mistakenly transported by this process in deference to the endogenous polyamines.

Lipophilic basic amines

Basic compounds having a lipophilic component are taken up by the lung probably by a combination of the mechanisms described above. It was found in lung perfusion models that basic amines with a $pK_a > 8.5$ were sequestered to a much greater degree than amines with $pK_a < 7.0$ [25, 26].

Fowler and co-worker later showed for a series of aliphatic amines that lung specificity was dependent on both the amino group and the lipophilicity of the alkyl group [27].

Similar results were obtained for the bronchodilator prodrug ibuterol ($pK_a = 9.1$) in the isolated, ventilated and perfused lung model; the lung uptake of the lipophilic prodrug was about 40 times higher than that of the very hydrophilic parent compound terbutaline [4].

Lung selectivity of bambuterol

As mentioned above, we had observed that some lipophilic ester prodrugs of terbutaline were efficiently taken up by the lung where they subsequently bioconverted to terbutaline [4]. However, their particular lung distribution properties could not be taken advantage of since these prodrugs were rapidly hydrolyzed to terbutaline already during the first-pass through the gut wall and the liver. On the other hand, bambuterol with its high hydrolytic stability could be expected to distribute to and be taken up by the lung.

When this was studied in a model using the isolated, perfused and ventilated guinea pig lung, it was found that bambuterol indeed was taken up by the lung, and that it together with its metabolites were concentrated by at least a factor 7 in the lung tissue relative to the perfusate [28]. Studies with terbutaline in a similar rat-model indicate an equal distribution between lung and perfusion medium [4]. Oxidative as well as hydrolytic metabolism of bambuterol took place in the lung tissue, since hydroxylated bambuterol (metabolite II) as well as the monocarbamate (metabolite III) together with traces of terbutaline were detected. The lung tissue retained the metabolites since only traces of them were detected in the perfusate. A tissue distribution study in mice showed that bambuterol has a very selective distribution to the lung also compared to other tissues such as skeletal muscle, the myocardium and the brain (Fig. 6).

The lung-to-plasma concentration ratio at 12 h, following a single

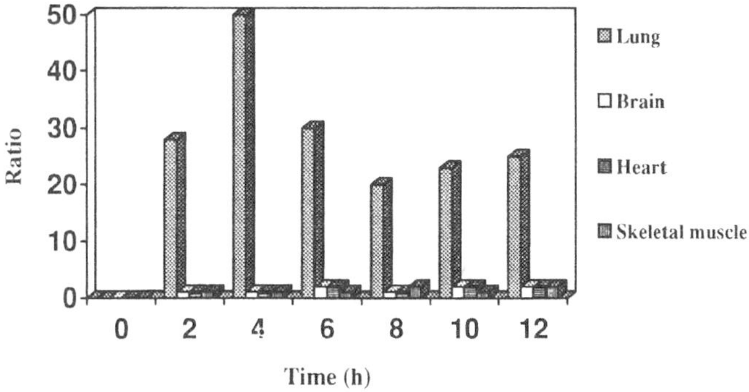

Fig. 6. Tissue to plasma concentration ratio of bambuterol after oral administration of 3H-bambuterol to mice

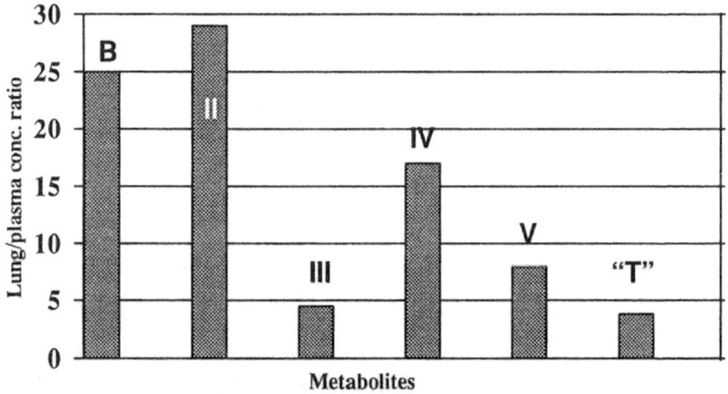

Fig. 7. Lung to plasma concentration ratios for bambuterol and some of its metabolites at 12 hours following oral administration of 3H-bambuterol to mice. For numbering, see Fig. 5

oral dose of the drug to mice, was about 25 for bambuterol itself. A lung-selective distribution was also found for several metabolites of bambuterol, and the terbutaline fraction displayed a lung-to-plasma concentration ratio of about 3.5 at 12h [29] (Fig. 7).

In this context, it should be remembered that even a small lung-to-plasma concentration ratio for terbutaline would give a beneficial effect-side effect ratio; for example, a ratio of 2 means that a therapeutic lung concentration can be obtained at half the usual plasma concentration of terbutaline, which would reduce the systemic side effects since they are proportional to the plasma concentration of active drug. If the same favorable distribution is found also in man, one should experience significantly less systemic side effects, such as tremor, in clinical studies when bambuterol is compared with other oral bronchodilators, in equi-bronchodilating doses.

Lung selectivity of bambuterol in patients?

Bambuterol was shown to be as effective as other oral bronchodilators in asthmatic patients, but a significantly lower incidence of tremor was generally observed. Could this be due to an enhanced distribution of terbutaline by bambuterol to the lung, as observed in animal studies?

One study was designed to try to answer this question [30]. The study was performed as a double-blind, multicentre trial with parallel group design with two randomized groups; one treated with bambuterol and the other with terbutaline controlled release (CR) tablets. The blinding was preserved by using a double-dummy technique. At the end of the run-in period, the patients were randomized into either the bambuterol (103 patients) or the terbutaline CR treatment group (102 patients). Within each group, every patient was given three different doses of the drug, calculated to give comparable plasma concentrations of terbutaline, (bambuterol: 5, 10 and 20 mg once nightly, terbutaline CR: 2, 4, and 8 mg b.i.d.) in three different periods of two weeks each in a randomized order. A wash-out period of one week was included between every treatment period.

The results from this dose-response study are presented in Fig. 8, where the effect, peak expiratory flow (PEF), and the side effect, tremor, measured as their differences between the treatment- and run-in periods (morning ΔPEF and Δtremor score) are depicted. Tremor increased with dose for both treatments, as expected, since it should be proportional to the plasma concentration of terbutaline, but tremor was significantly lower for bambuterol at equipotent bronchodilating dose. Even if only the ΔPEF for the lowest doses differed significantly, the morning ΔPEF for terbutaline CR increased linearely with dose, while morning ΔPEF for bambuterol showed a more shallow appearance. This

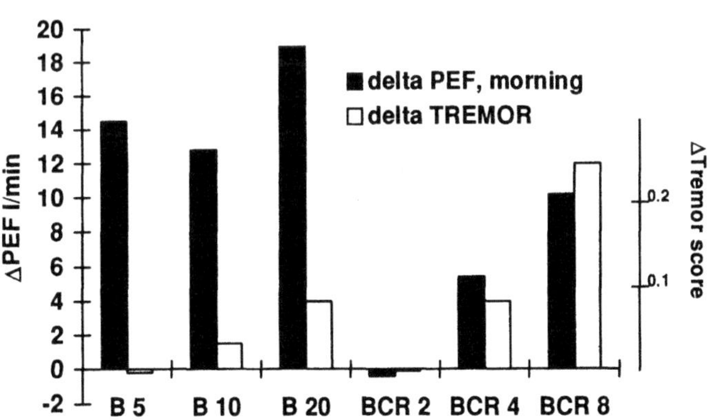

Fig. 8. Bambuterol - terbutaline CR dose-response study

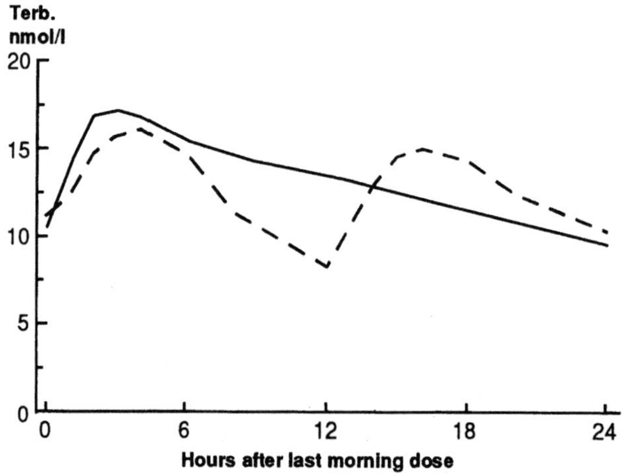

Fig. 9. Steady-state terbutaline plasma concentrations after bambuterol 20 mg once daily (solid line), and terbutaline CR, 7.5 mg b.i.d., (broken line). Mean values from 18 healthy subjects

indicates, but does not prove, that terbutaline generated from bambuterol might be more efficiently utilized than when terbutaline is slowly absorbed from a CR tablet.

Another explanation for the lower incidence of tremor could be the smooth plasma concentration profile of terbutaline generated from bambuterol compared to terbutaline CR (see Fig. 9).

Human pharmacokinetics

Bambec® produces steady-state plasma concentrations of terbutaline with little fluctuation. During once-daily dosage, the ratio between peak and trough concentrations is usually equal to or lower than 2.0 (15). Terbutaline concentrations increase linearly with dose. Figure 9 shows that bambuterol given once daily competes favourably with terbutaline in controlled-release tablets given twice daily (Astra Draco, data on file).

The reason for the sustained plasma concentrations of terbutaline generated from bambuterol is threefold:

- Bambuterol is absorbed for a long time from the gastro-intestinal tract.
- The production of terbutaline by oxidation and hydrolysis is slow and continuous.
- The elimination of terbutaline by renal excretion and metabolic inactivation is slow in itself.

Clinical experience

In clinical studies evaluated thus far, bambuterol tablets once daily has been given to more than 2000 asthmatic patients from the age of 16 to 82 years. The result obtained show that:

- Bambec® is an effective bronchodilator with 24 hours duration of action in the maintenance treatment of asthma, particularly nocturnal asthma.
- Bambec® reduces diurnal variation in lung function.
- The dosage of Bambec® is 10 to 20 mg once daily. There is evidence that Bambec® is most effective in patients with more severe disease.
- Bambec® (once daily) is at least as effective as oral terbutaline CR, salbutamol CR and theophylline CR (twice daily), and oral terbutaline and salbutamol (t.i.d.) in the maintenance treatment of asthma.
- Bambec® 10 or 20 mg once daily produced similar levels of bronchodilation inchildren, adult and elderly patients.
- Bambec® induced improvements in lung function have been maintained for periods more than 4 years in the long-term management of patients with chronic reversible obstructive airways disease.
- Bambec® 20 mg at bedtime and inhaled salmeterol 50 µg bid, in a group of moderate to severe asthmatic patients, showed similar efficacy in control of nocturnal and daily symptoms of asthma.
- Bambec® has a lower frequency and severity of adverse events as compared with other oral bronchodilators in equi-bronchodilating doses.

Conclusions

Bambec® is a new long-acting β_2-agonist in asthma therapy which offers a unique advantage – a once daily oral regimen which gives reliable bronchodilation throughout the 24 hours.

The pharmacodynamic effect is achieved because bambuterol is slowly absorbed, and then metabolized to its active principle, terbutaline. Over the 24 hours between doses, terbutaline levels remain steadily within a narrow range, avoiding extreme peaks and troughs.

These pharmacokinetics do not only favour prolonged relief from asthmatic symptoms, but also help to reduce systemic, sympathomimetic adverse effects such as tremor.

Bambec®, which is given as an evening dose, is particularly suited to preventing early morning asthma attacks, a most troublesome problem for patients with asthma.

References

1. Bauer CA, Svenson L-Å (1992) Bambuterol (Bambec®): A new long-acting oral bronchodilator. Drugs of Today 28: 547–557
2. Kristoffersson J, Svensson L-Å, Tegnér K (1974) Drug latentiation of terbutaline. In vitro serum esterase catalyzed hydrolysis of a series of acyl-substituded mono- and diesters of terbutaline. Acta Pharm Suec 11: 427–438
3. Hörnblad Y, Ripe E, Magnusson PO, Tegnér K (1976) The metabolic and clinical activity of terbutaline and its ester prodrug ibuterol. Eur J Clin Pharmacol 10: 9–18
4. Ryrfeldt Å, Nilsson E (1978) Uptake and biotransformation of ibuterol and terbutaline in isolated perfused rat and guinea pig lungs. Biochem Pharmacol 27: 301–305
5. Svensson L-Å (1987) Development of β_2-adrenoceptor agonist bronchodilator prodrugs. In: Hollinger MA (ed) Current topics in pulmonary pharmacology and toxicology, Vol. 3. Elsevier, New York, 1–26
6. Olsson OAT, Svensson L-Å (1984) New lipophilic terbutaline ester prodrugs with long effect duration. Pharm Res 1: 19–23
7. Svensson L-Å (1991) A prodrug approach to a long-acting β_2-agonist. DN&P 4: 544–549
8. Tunek A, Svensson L-Å (1988) Bambuterol, a carbamate ester prodrug of

terbutaline, as inhibitor of cholinesterases in human blood. Drug Metab Dispos 16: 759–764
9. Sharma M, Svensson L-Å (1991) Bambuterol, a selective inhibitor of plasma butyryl cholinesterase. In: Massoulié J et al (eds) Cholinesterases. Structure, function, mechanism, genetics, and cell biology. ACS Books, Washington, DC
10. Wetterlin K (1972) Resolution of terbutaline, a new β-sympathomimetic amine. J Med Chem 15: 1182–1183
11. Jeppsson A-B, Johansson U, Waldeck B (1984) Steric aspects of agonism and antagonism at β-adrenoceptors: Experiments with the enantiomers of terbutaline and pindolol. Acta Pharmacol et toxicol 54: 285–291
12. Tunek A, Kennedy B-M, Svensson L-Å (1991) Stereoselective interactions of bambuterol with human plasma cholinesterase. Symposium on recent progress in extrahepatic metabolism (May 15–17, Ronneby) Abst 19
13. Lindberg C, Roos C, Tunek A, Svensson L-Å (1989) Metabolism of bambuterol in rat liver microsomes: Identification of hydroxylated and demethylated products by liquid chromatography mass spectrometry. Drug Metab Disp 17: 311–322
14. Svensson L-Å, Tunek A (1988) The design and bioactivation of presystemically stable prodrugs. Drug Metab Rev 19: 165–194
15. Svensson L-Å (1987) Bambuterol- a prodrug-prodrug with built-in hydrolysis brake. Acta Pharm Suec 24: 333–341
16. Tunek A, Borgström L, Nyberg L (1986) Metabolism in man of ^{3}H-bambuterol: A carbamate ester prodrug of terbutaline. Acta Pharmacol Toxicol 59 [Suppl 5]: 214
17. Viby Mogensen J, Bang U, Nyberg L, Weibull E, Nilsson M (Manuscript in preparation)
18. Tunek A, Hjertberg E, Viby Mogensen J (1991) Interactions of bambuterol with human serum cholinesterase of the genotypes E_uE_u (normal), E_aE_a (atypical) and E_uE_a. Biochem Pharmacol 41: 345–348
19. Yata N, Toyoda T, Murakami T, Nishiura A, Higashi Y (1990) Phosphatidylserine as a determinant for the tissue distribution of weakly basic drugs in rats. Pharm Res 7: 1019–1025
20. Nishiura A, Murakami T, Higashi Y, Yata N (1988) Role of phosphatidylserine in the cellular and subcellular lung distribution of quinidine in rats. Pharm Res 5: 209–213
21. Yoshida H, Kamiya A, Okumura K, Hori R (1989) Contribution of monoamine oxidase (MAO) to the binding of tertiaty basic drugs in lung mitochondria. Pharm Res 6: 877–882
22. Ishida H, Okumura K, Hori R (1990) Contribution of monoamine oxidase (MAO) to the binding of tertiary basic drugs in isolated perfused rat lung. Pharm Res 7: 398–401
23. Reasor MJ, Koshut RA, Castranova V (1979) Biochemical characteristics

of rat alveolar macrophages with chlorophentermine-induced phospholipidosis: Variations with increased cell size. Exp Mol Pathol 31: 297–307
24. Smith LL (1985) The identification and characterization of a polyamine-accumulating system in the lung. Biochem Soc Trans 13: 332–334
25. Anderson MW, Orton TC, Picket RD, Eling TE (1974) Accumulation of amines in the isolated perfused rabbit lung. J Pharmacol Exp Ther 189: 456–466
26. Orton TC, Anderson MW, Picket RD, Eling TE, Fouts JR (1973) Xenobiotic accumulation and metabolism by isolated perfused rabbit lung. J Pharmacol Exp Ther 186: 482–487
27. Fowler JS, Gallagher BM, MacGregor RR, Wolf AP (1976) Carbon-11 labeled aliphatic amines in lung uptake and metabolism studies: potential for dynamic measurements in vivo. J Pharmacol Exp Ther 198: 133–145
28. Ryrfeldt Å, Nilsson E, Tunek A, Svensson L-Å (1988) Bambuterol: Uptake and metabolism in guinea pig isolated lungs. Pharm Res 5: 151–155
29. Levin E, Tegnér K (Manuscript in preparation)
30. Gnosspelius Y, Olsson H (Manuscript in preparation)

Correspondence: Prof. Dr. Leif-Ake Svensson, Department of Medicinal Chemistry, Astra Draco AB, Box 34, S-22100 Lund, Sweden.

Discussion

Dr. Kummer: Thank you indeed, Dr. Svensson, for this presentation of how a fast-acting drug was converted into an orally acting long-acting drug.

As you know, most people today prefer topic treatment with inhaled drugs, but I thought it would be justified to hear more about this prodrug concept that you have developed for terbutaline.

Dr. Ulmer: Dr. Svensson, you showed us that you have less side effects with bambuterol than with terbutaline.

Dr. Svensson: Yes.

Dr. Ulmer: Maybe, when you give a puff, you get a short, steep increase of blood concentration and it comes down very fast. So the duration of the side effects may be shorter with your short-acting agent. But if you have high concentration for a prolonged period, does this not create a problem?

Dr. Svensson: Bambuterol is a tablet with 24 hours' duration of action. We really have no plasma concentration peak. The peak-trough value is usually below 2. So it is a very smooth plasma concentration profile. But even when you use controlled-release formulations of different bronchodilators, such as salbutamol and terbutaline, where you also have rather smooth plasma concentration profiles, bambuterol still gives significantly less side effects.

NN: What about long-term side effects?

Dr. Svensson: Well, we don't see any, and after a week tremor usually disappears due to tachyphylaxis.

Dr. Johnson: One of the problems about the prodrug approach is the incidence of poor metabolizers of these prodrugs. Have you looked at all whether there are any genetic polymorphisms in the metabolic routes from bambuterol to terbutaline, and what the incidence is likely to be in the asthmatic population?

Dr. Svensson: We have looked at the different groups of patients, those having impaired plasma cholinesterase activity, and those having an impaired oxidative metabolism. I showed data demonstrating that patients having the atypical gene for plasma cholinesterase are able to generate the same amount of terbutaline from bambuterol as normal individuals. We have also found that even if there is a variation in the oxidative metabolism of bambuterol, the variation in the end product terbutaline is small, because hydrolysis and oxidation may compensate for each other.

Dr. Kummer: This is something that I wonder, that people are just fond of one particular drug and respond beautifully and others don't. So I think it's an appropriate endeavour to line out the different drugs to our better knowledge. So we don't get stuck with one drug and get all desperate if the patient doesn't respond. So we change him over to another one, maybe the patient is much more grateful. But I think these clinical questions will be dealt in detail tomorrow by Dr. Selroos, who will give a comparison between salmeterol and bambuterol.

Dr. Lichtenschopf (Weyer): I have a question, not only to bambuterol but to all long-acting drugs. When salmeterol came to Austria in the year 1992, it was supposed to have an anti-inflammatory activity. In the year 1993, some researchers denied this. What can you say about the anti-inflammatory activity of long-acting drugs, particularly of bambuterol?

Dr. Svensson: This is a very tough question.

Dr. Kummer: Can I bridge this by changing the term into "modulating inflammation". Not just purely anti-inflammatory. That is probably too strong a term. But are there any data on the modulation of inflammatory mediators?

Dr. Svensson: Of course, you can show in different animal models in vitro and in vivo that many beta-agonists, not only the long-acting ones, have some sort of anti-inflammatory effects. But when it comes to the clinic, I doubt that there is any hard data showing that these drugs really have an anti-inflammatory effect. I guess you also should be careful so you don't forget to give the patients the corticosteroids.

Dr. Johnson: Just a comment about the anti-inflammatory point. I think you were quite right to change the term, because when we became interested in the pharmacological and the animal data that these types of drugs would have this sort of activity, the difficulty was that people began to assume anti-inflammatory equalled corticosteroid-like action. These drugs would never have that sort of effect. But I think we are seeing now some clinical data that may be teaching us a little bit more about inflammation as well as what these drugs can do and can't do. There is evidence in man, albeit in the nose that salmeterol will block vascular permeability to histamine and antigen challenge in human subjects. After one week's treatment you can show an effect on broncho-alveolar lavage eosinophil activation. And there is data showing that after two months' treatment in asthmatic patients, the activation status of inflammatory cells in the airways is decreased on salmeterol compared to placebo. And so I think the difficulty was that the term was inappropriately used at the beginning, and I think we must carry on using steroids, but it might be that these other drugs do have some minor inflammatory modulating activity. Whether that is clinically important I think is the key question and that requires more study.

Dr. Ulmer: You need the liver for your drug to work. What happens to patients who have liver problems?

Dr. Svensson: You are right. People with severe liver problems should not take bambuterol. They should be given terbutaline instead.

Development of β_2-receptors in infancy and childhood

M. Götz

Department of Paediatric and Adolescent Medicine, Wilhelminenspital, Vienna, Austria

Summary

At birth, intraalveolar fluid is rapidly displaced by air and excessive interstitial fluid is absorbed into the vascular system. This removal of fluid and surfactant release are presumed to be linked to pulmonary β-adrenergic stimulation. Administration of β-blockers to fetal lambs was shown to abolish the increase in surfactant release that normally accompanies labour and delivery. Similar observations have been reported in fetal rabbits. Little is known about the development of receptors in humans. Indirect evidence from functional studies in human babies suggest similar changes although the ontogeny of human pulmonary receptors remains largely unknown. During gestation both neural and non-neural receptor types change. With advancing gestational age the number of intrapulmonary β-adrenergic receptors increases nearly tenfold between the 15th gestational week and term. Receptor distribution shows a predominance in alveolar walls, bronchiolar and bronchial walls and in airway smooth muscle. It has been shown both in vitro and in vivo that exogenous glucocorticoid increases pulmonary β-receptors. Thus, glucocorticoids may be responsible for the increased pulmonary β-receptor concentration in late gestation. Glucocorticoids may increase β-adrenergic reponsiveness by both changes in receptor concentration and coupling of receptor occupancy to response.

Postnatally, several early studies failed to find bronchodilator responses to nebulized β_2-agonists in infancy. It was therefore believed for many years that β-agonists were ineffective in this age group. Recent well designed studies have however shown significant bronchodilator effects and protection against bronchoconstricting agents. Clinical improvements were shown both for infants treated with β_2-agents alone or in combination with steroids. Methodological aspects may be one reason for discrepancies between older and more recent data concerning bronchodilatation. It therefore seems that infants have functioning β_2-receptors from birth and that stimulation of these receptors produces the same effect as in older children. Clinically, the response is often quite small and interindividual differences are seen. Preschool children show the same response to β_2-adrenergic agents as do schoolchildren.

Prenatal β-adrenergic receptor development

Uncomplicated birth is linked to normal commencement of gas exchange. Surfactant release and removal of intraalveolar fluid are the two most important steps towards this. Stimulation of β-adrenergic receptors seems to initiate these vital changes [1]. In humans, very little data is available on prenatal receptor function. Thus virtually all information is derived from animal work. In fetal lambs, administration of β-blocking agents such as propranolol was shown to diminish the tracheal fluid flow [2] whereas surfactant release from alveolar type II cells [3] which normally accompanies labour and delivery was increased by β-adrenergic agents. In addition to demonstration in vitro of increased surfactant synthesis by β-adrenergic substances [4], terbutaline, a β-adrenergic agonist, was shown to stimulate surfactant phospholipid secretion in a concentration dependent way in both undifferentiated and differentiated fetal type II cells [5]. It should be remembered that alveolar type II cells make up only 5 to 7 percent of the total alveolar cell population and that receptor density is relatively low on these cells.

Airway smooth muscle, from the trachea to the terminal bronchioles, contains significant numbers of β-adrenergic receptors, and density increases with decreasing airway size [6]. These receptors are almost entirely of the β2 subtype in humans. Smooth muscle in the developing lung matures rapidly soon after it differentiates from the mesenchyme. Fetal pigs, weighing 8–10 g during their pseudoglandular phase, showed airway narrowing indicating functional innervation following electrical stimulation and acetylcholine action [7]. Indirect evidence from functional studies in human babies suggest similar changes although the ontogeny of human pulmonary receptors remains largely unknown. Infants born by caesarean section are more prone to respiratory difficulties suggesting lack of catecholamines induced by labour. Although acute administration of β-adrenergics may reduce respiratory hazards in the newborn, chronic use of β-adrenergic substances during pregnancy may increase respiratory difficulties in the newborn. This may be evidence for β-adrenergic receptor downregulation [1].

During gestation both neural and non-neural receptor types change. With advancing gestational age the number of intrapulmonary β-adrenergic receptors increases nearly tenfold between the 14th week of gestation and term [8]. In rats disproportionately higher specific grain densities over alveolar lining cells could be seen in 3-months-old rats in comparison to 1-day-old aminals [9]. In rabbits, airways and alveoli contain β-adrenoreceptors with airway containing more than alveoli both in fetal and adult lung. After glucocorticoid treatment there is preferential increase in fetal alveolar β-adrenoreceptors. This increase is consistent with a maturational effect of glucocorticoid treatment on fetal alveolar function [10]. In fetal pigs, inhibition of airway narrowing by β-adrenoceptor agonists could be achieved from the main stem bronchi to terminal regions of late generation branches (20–35 μp) as evidence of β-receptors in the smooth muscle at 44–48 days of gestation [7]. Beta-adrenergic receptors have been mapped by autoradiography using radiolabelled beta-adrenergic antagonists to alveolar walls, airway and vascular smooth muscle, submucosal glands and airway epithelium [11]. An excellent review of developmental aspects of the neural control of the lung is provided by Davis and Kercsmar [12].

Bronchomotor tone and associated spontaneous activity, which moves fluid along the airways, may serve to maintain positive airway pressure and thus to support the stimulus necessary for continued growth of the lung. Draining off of positive pressure will result in a hypoplastic lung [7].

Beta-adrenergic function and presence of β-receptors develops early, probably parallel with cholinergic function and development of cholinergic innervation. It has been shown both in vitro and in vivo that exogenous glucocorticoid increases pulmonary β-receptors selectively whereas other organ systems are not influenced [6]. Thus glucocorticoids may be responsible for the increased pulmonary β-receptor concentration in late gestation. As a consequence sensitivity of receptors increases dramatically towards the end of gestation. The role of endogenous catecholamines in adrenergic receptor development and functional maturation remains to be elucidated. If there is a role it would explain decreased respiratory problems when delivery occurs with labour, with increased adrenergic stimulation or after administration of glucocorticoids.

Function of β_2-adrenergic receptors and problem orientation

Generally, functions of β_2-receptors are best summarized as smooth muscle relaxation, mast cell mediator release inhibition, reduction of permeability of small bronchial vessels, increase of ephithelial fluid transport, increase of submucosal gland secretion (together with β_1-adrenoceptors) and activity on alveolar type II cells. There is no doubt that in humans β_2-adrenergic receptors are present at birth. As mentioned, intraalveolar fluid removal and surfactant efflux are stimulated by β_2-adrenergic activity. When immediate bronchodilatation is later required, smooth muscle relaxation is of the greatest importance. In young children endothelial tightening and fluid removal may be of equal importance in overcoming bronchial obstruction.

Treatment of asthma and other wheezing disorders in the early age group is difficult and the role of β_2-adrenergic agents has been judged variably. Furthermore concern followed reports of increased asthma mortality seen in New Zealand in the 80s [13]. Changes in asthma severity, prescribing habits, product specificity and epidemiologic background have all been implicated. Much of the evidence provided has remained circumstantial and causal relationships are still far from clear. Even recent data from Canada linking increased bronchodilator use and increased death or near death fail to resolve these urgent questions [15]. Regardless of whether β-agonists are directly responsible for adverse effects or are simply a marker for more severe asthma, heavy use of these agents should alert clinicians that it is necessary to reevaluate the patients' conditions [14]. Although this β-agonist dilemma [15] cannot be directly extrapolated to infants and children it is evident that safety considerations when using β-adrenergic bronchodilators are relevant and should be borne in mind whenever prolonged use of β_2-agents is considered [16]. It is clear that in paediatrics adverse effects of β_2-adrenergic agents are conceivable. They consist of overreliance on these drugs at the expense of prophylaxis, neglect of cardiovascular effects, downregulation of β_2-receptors, and increased bronchial responsiveness.

Use of bronchodilators in wheezy infants

Wheezing in infants may be caused by numerous conditions including bronchiolitis, asthma, cystic fibrosis, gasto-oesophageal reflux, aspiration, structural defects and several others. Wheezing triggered by viral infection as a forerunner to later asthma is but one aspect of the whole spectrum of wheezing illnesses [17]. The younger the child, particularly below age 5, the greater the possibility of an alternative diagnosis to asthma for recurrent wheeze. Fortunately, the majority of infants with wheezing have transient conditions associated with diminished airway function at birth and do not have increased risks of asthma or allergies later in life [18]. In a substantial minority however, wheezing episodes are probably related to a predisposition for asthma. Whereas the role of β_2-agonists remains undisputed in relieving acute bronchospasm [19] and as drugs of choice for infrequent episodic asthma in preschool and schoolchildren [20] treatment of wheezy infants with bronchodilators continues to be an unresolved question. In view of the fact that hospital admissions of wheezing children up to the age of four years has increased fourfold over the last two decades [21] clear answers as to the drugs' benefit would be welcome.

While older reports fail to demonstrate effects of beta-adrenergic bronchodilators [22, 23] the majority of recent data suggest beneficial effects from aerosolized medication when adequate doses are used (salbutamol 0.15–0.3 mg/kg). Thus, in children less than two years of age, two doses of salbutamol administered with an interval of one hour, resulted in significant reduction of wheezing and improved oxygen saturation in the emergency unit [24]. Beneficial effects were also seen in preterm infants with respiratory symptoms, spontaneously breathing wheezing infants [25], and ventilator-dependent premature babies [26]. In addition, Kraemer et al. [27] were able to show significantly improved lung function in infants aged 2 to 18 months with bronchopulmonary dysplasia. Use of a babyhaler showed that 57.1 % of patients responded after 400 μg and 92.9 % after use of 600 μg.

In comparison to placebo clinically significant improvements in bronchiolitic young children aged 1 to 21 months were seen with a maximum benefit after 30 minutes [28]. Unfortunately, effects were short-lived and were no longer demonstrable by 60 minutes. Although salbutamol was safe and efficacious the clinical relevance of these findings is somewhat questionable.

Clinically, a trial of β_2-agents seems to be warranted in any case with significant wheezing [17] and respiratory distress. Infants requiring β_2-agonist treatment consistently more frequently than three times per week should be given more conventional long-term asthma therapy [29]. The clinically quite variable response to β-adrenergic drugs is not caused by absence of receptors but may be explained by functional immaturity. However desirable physiologic data to support and confirm responses would be it does not seem justified to subject all patients thus treated to infant lung function festing. In addition, cost factors and availability of measurements must be taken into account. A clinical score to assess wheezing has been suggested [30] which has the benefit of very good interobserver reliability (Table 1). It ought thus be more widely acceptable that clinical improvements are equally important as functional data. Functional maturity of β_2-adrenergic receptors in infants has been questioned for many years solely on the basis of failure to improve lung function.

Table 1. Clinical assessment of respiratory distress in wheezing infants

	Points					
	0	1	2	3	4	maximum
Wheezing						
Expiration	none	end	one half	three fourths	all	4
Inspiration	none	part	all			2
Location	none	< 2 of 4 lung fields	> 3 of lung fields			2
Retractions						
Supraclavicular	none	mild	moderate	marked		3
Intercostal	none	mild	moderate	marked		3
Subcostal	none	mild	moderate	marked		3
Total						17

Adapted from Lowell [30]

Use of inhaled β_2-agents is further complicated by unresolved issues relating to bronchial responsiveness in newborn and young infants. Recent evidence suggests that bronchial responsiveness in this age group may be increased compared to older children [31]. In this context presence of functional β-adrenergic receptors in the airways of infants was demonstrated by reversal of histamine induced bronchoconstriction during the first 12 months of life [32] (Fig. 1). The considerable inter-individual variation of observed responses may explain clinical differences alluded to above. These differences may also be based on receptor polymorphism. Already earlier, Tepper [33] showed responses of infants aged around 3.5 months both to methacholine and to metaproterenol indicating properly functioning response patterns (Fig. 2). Interestingly, bronchial sensitivity to inhaled histamine in healthy, nonatopic children was also found to be much higher than expected from surveys in adults [34]. Whether these data provide evidence that during infancy and childhood bronchial reactivity is higher than previously assumed must remain speculative. Why in light of the increased infantile and childhood bronchial responsiveness β_2-agents should be of uncertain effectiveness remains open and suggests that alternative mechanisms

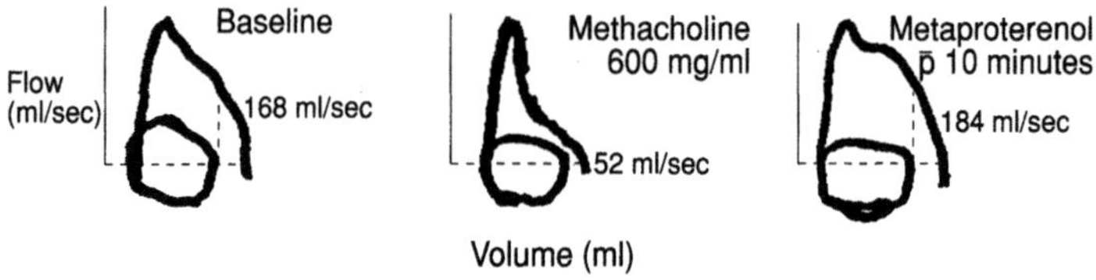

Fig. 1. Change in partial expiratory flow curve and maximal expiratory flow at FRC from baseline to completion of methacholine challenge and 10 min after inhalation of metaproterenol
3.5 mo; 59 cm; (Tepper, ref. 33)

may play a role. Osmolality and pH of inhaled bronchodilator solutions may be of importance. Aerosol acidity may induce hypoxaemia shortly after aerosol administration but this is not normally associated with untoward clinical side effects or deterioration of lung function [35]. Increases of thoracic gas volume and airway resistance were seen when wet inhalations were used. Baseline lung function may be an important factor contributing to drug response as may be age at birth and perhaps, to a lesser degree, viral infections and atopy. Finally, in this age group mucus and mucosal oedema are of more importance than smooth

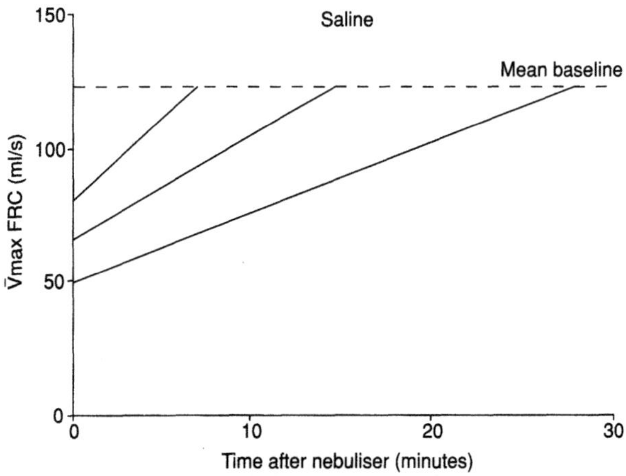

Fig. 2. Effect of salbutamol on histamine induced bronchoconstriction in healthy infants (Henderson et al., ref. 32)

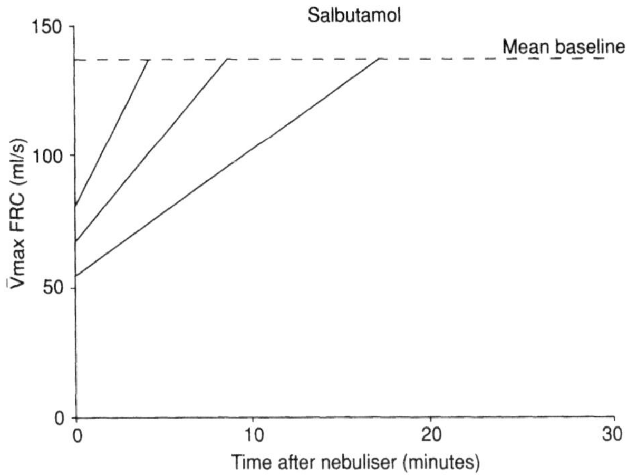

Fig. 3. Recovery following histamine induced bronchoconstriction in infants who received saline or salbutamol

muscle contraction. These changes may be considered evidence of ongoing airway inflammation of early onset.

Fiberoptic investigations will show whether airway morphology is actually altered at an early stage already. Presently, technical and ethical considerations preclude wide application of this technique. Indirect evidence in adults suggests upregulation of IL-6 and IL-8 expression as evidence of ongoing inflammation. It is possible that β-adrenergic agonists suppress both synthesis and secretion of proinflammatory interleukins (Block L-H, unpublished data). In children, monitoring of these interleukins peripherally would be an ideal means to assess staging of inflammation and response to treatment. At present monitoring of eosinophil activity seems an available and promising alternative [36]. Overall, present data suggest good if somewhat unpredictable effectiveness of β_2-agonists in the early age group and reduction of airway obstruction irrespective of the underlying mechanisms.

Certainly one of the most important mechanisms of β_2-adrenergic effectiveness is maintenance of mucociliary transport. Beta-adrenergic agonists act on beta-adrenergic receptors in airway epithelial cells and stimulate chloride ion secretion and therefore water secretion [37].

Periciliary fluid characteristics are clearly important for removal of secretions.

At present there is no evidence that in the early years of life prolonged use of β_2-adrenergic agents increases bronchial responsiveness as has been observed in the older age groups [38].

In viral bronchiolitis, individualized β-agent administration should be followed and when non-responsiveness has been established clinically β_2-adrenergic therapy should not be continued. The trial period time is not clearly defined but the author's impression would be not to continue monotherapy for more than 24 hours. In general, use of β-adrenergic agents for bronchiolitis has been disappointing [39].

Drug administration in the first years of life may be difficult. There is a paucity of suitably designed and tested inhaler devices specific for the age group 0–2 years. Compressor driven aerosols have now been largely replaced by metered dose inhalers and large volume chambers (spacers) fitted with face masks. Drug doses thus actually reaching the lungs are small however and may be as little as 2 % whilst the majority of drugs becomes trapped in the spacer. These results may indicate that higher doses than the current recommendations may be required to actually be effective in the lungs [40]. Although it is generally accepted that inhaled drugs should be used preferentially [41] more drug is delivered by nebulizers i.e. 2.5 times higher than the dose applied by spacers [29].

Use of β_2-agonists in older children

Beta-$_2$ adrenergic substances have lost their predominant use in long-term management of asthma since evidence of deterioration of bronchial hyperresponsiveness or clinical stabilization emerged both in adults [42] and in children [38, 43]. Sporadic and single drug use is warranted in acute or infrequent asthma where their superior activity remains undisputed. Even continuous salbutamol nebulization was found safe and efficacious in children with status asthmaticus [44]. In adults, even in patients considered by their family physicians to have such mild asthma that inhaled corticosteroids would not provide clinical benefit, low doses of budesonide produced striking improvements in both symptom control and airway obstruction [45]. It may clearly be worth investigating similar aspects in older children with the goal of evading development of airway inflammation.

Short-term infusions of salbutamol have been shown to curtail the progression of acute asthma without clinically significant side-effects [45]. Spacers are the preferred method of application and are equally effective as nebulizers to deliver β_2-agonists in acute asthma in preschool and schoolchildren [47].

Inhaled long acting β_2-agents such as salmeterol and formoterol have been assessed in children [48]. Indications generally are primarily activity induced asthma [49] and night time wheezing. In addition replacement of continuous short-acting β_2-agents by long-acting substances should be undertaken when continued or prolonged use of these substances are considered [50]. As a cautionary note one should remember that long-acting β_2-adrenergic substances should be used only in conjunction with anti-inflammatory treatments, where they were shown to significantly improve peak flows and reduce symptoms [51].

Desensitization of the agonist mediated response does occur after prolonged or repeated exposure to β-adrenergic medication in a dose dependent fashion and is more pronounced in mature than in immature (rabbit) airways [52]. Concerns relating to reduced responsiveness to bronchodilators as seen in adults may be of importance [53]. In the same line, development of subsensitivity to salbutamol after continuous exposure to salmeterol thus requiring higher doses of salbutamol relief medication was reported [54]. Longer term use even once daily only may lead to waning of bronchoprotective effects against exercise induced asthma as was shown recently in a 2 x 28 days crossover study using salmeterol in schoolchildren [55].

In conclusion, β_2-adrenergic receptors are present at birth. Beta-adrenergic agents elicit an unpredictable effect in the newborn and infant period. They should still be tried in the various wheezing conditions of this age group. Alternative or complementary drugs such as inhaled corticosteroids show efficacy on a long-term basis but require careful monitoring [56]. As efficacious bronchodilators in the older age groups β-adrenergic agents have remained unchallenged. Whether newer long-acting β-agents will secure a firm place in childhood asthma remains to be determined but seems likely.

References

1. Roberts JM, Jacobs MM, Cheng JB et al (1985) Fetal pulmonary β-adrenergic receptors: Characterization in the human and in vitro modulation by glucocorticoids in the rabbit. Pediatr Pulmonol 1 [Suppl]: S 69–S 76
2. Walters DV, Olver RE (1978) The role of catecholamines in lung liquid absorption at birth. Pediatr Res 12: 239–43
3. Oyarzun MF, Clements JA (1978) Control of lung surfactant by ventilation, adrenergic mediators, and prostaglandins in the rabbit. Am Rev Respir Dis 117: 879–91
4. Mettler NR, Gay ME, Schuffman S et al (1981) Beta-adrenergic induced synthesis and secretion of phosphatydilcholine by isolated pulmonary type II cells. Lab Invest 45: 575–80
5. Kresch MJ, Lima DM, Lu H (1996) Developmental regulation of phospholipid secretion by fetal type II pneumocytes. Biochim Biophys Acta 1299: 39–46
6. Barnes PJ, Basbaum CB (1983) Mapping of adrenergic receptors in the trachea by autoradiography. Exp Lung Res 5: 183–92
7. Sparrow MP, Warwick SP, Mitchell HP (1994) Foetal airway motor tone in prenatal lung development of the pig. Eur Respir J 7: 1416–24
8. Barnes PJ, Karliner JS, Dollery CT (1980) Human lung adrenoceptors studied by radioligand binding. Clin Sci 58: 457–62
9. Schell N, Durham D, Murphree SS et al (1992) Ontogeny of β-adrenergic receptors in pulmonary arterial smooth muscle, bronchial smooth muscle, and alveolar lining cells in the rat. Am J Respir Cell Mol Biol 7: 317–24
10. Barnes P, Jacobs M, Roberts JM (1984) Glucocorticoids preferentially increase fetal alveolar β-adrenoceptors: autoradiographic evidence. Pediatr Res 18: 1191–4
11. Carstairs JS, Nimmo AJ, Barnes PJ (1985) Autoradiographic visualization of beta-adrenergic subtypes in human lung. Am Rev Respir Dis 132: 541–7
12. Davis PB, Kercsmar CM (1991) Neural control of the lung. In: Chernick V, Mellins RB (eds) Basic mechanisms of pediatric respiratory disease: cellular and integrative. BC Becker: Philadelphia, 203–20
13. Crane J, Pearce N, Flatt A et al (1989) Prescribed fenoterol and death from asthma in New Zealand 1981–1983: case-control study. Lancet i: 917–22
14. Spitzer WO, Suissa S, Ernst P et al (1992) The use of β-agonists and the risk of death and near death from asthma. N Engl J Med 326: 501–6
15. Burrows B, Lebowitz MD (1992) The β-agonist dilemma. N Engl J Med 326: 560–61
16. Eggleston PA (1997) Are β-adrenergic bronchodilators safe? Pediatrics 99: 729–30

17. Wilson NM (1989) Wheezy bronchitis revisited. Arch Dis Child 64: 1194–99
18. Martinez FD, Wright AL, Taussig LM et al (1995) Asthma and wheezing in the first six years of life. N Engl J Med 332: 133–8
19. Schuh S, Reider MJ, Canny G et al (1990) Nebulized albuterol in acute childhood asthma: Comparison of two doses. Pediatrics 86: 509–13
20. Warner JO, Neijens JH, Landau LI et al (1992) Asthma: a follow-up statement from an International Paediatric Asthma Consensus Group. Arch Dis Child 67: 240–8
21. Clough JB (1993) Bronchodilators in infancy. Thorax 48: 308
22. Lenney W, Milner AD (1978) At what age do bronchodilator drugs work? Arch Dis Child 53: 532–5
23. Silverman M (1984) Bronchodilators for wheezy infants? Arch Dis Child 59: 84–7
24. Bentur I, Canny GJ, Shields MD et al (1992) Controlled trial of nebulized albuterol in children younger than 2 years of age with acute asthma. Pediatrics 89: 133–7
25. Kraemer R, Frey U, Sommer CW et al (1991) Short-term effect of albuterol, delivered via a new auxiliary device, in wheezy infants. Am Rev Respir Dis 144: 347–51
26. Denjean A, Guimaraes H, Migdal M et al (1992) Dose-related bronchodilator response to aerosolized salbutamol (albuterol) in ventilator-dependent infants. J Pediatr 120: 974–9
27. Kraemer R, Birrer P, Modelska K et al (1992) A new baby-spacer device for aerosolized bronchodilator administration in infants with bronchopulmonary diseases. Eur J Pediatr 151: 57–60
28. Klassen TP, Rowe PC, Sutcliffe T et al (1991) Randomized trial of salbutamol in acute bronchiolitis. J Pediatr 118: 807–11
29. Global initiative for asthma (1995) Global strategy for asthma management and prevention NHLBI/WHO workshop report. National Institutes of Health Publication No 95-3659
30. Lowell DI, Lister G, von Koss H et al (1987) Wheezing in infants: the response to epinephrine. Pediatrics 79: 939–45
31. Montgomery GL, Tepper RS (1990) Changes in airway reactivity with age in normal infants and young children. Am Rev Respir Dis 142: 1372–5
32. Henderson AJW, Young S, Stick SM et al (1993) Effect of salbutamol on histamine induced bronchoconstriction in healthy infants. Thorax 48: 317–23
33. Tepper RS (1987) Airway reactivity in infants: a positive response to methacholine and metaproterenol. J Appl Physiol 62: 1155–9
34. Riedel F, von der Hardt H (1986) Bronchial sensitivity to inhaled histamine in healthy, nonatopic children. Pediatr Pulmonol 2: 15–8

35. Seidenburg J, Mir Y, von der Hardt H (1991) Hypoxaemia after nebulized salbutamol in wheezy infants: the importance of aerosol acidity. Arch Dis Child 66: 672–5
36. Koller DY, Herouy Y, Götz M et al (1995) Clinical value of monitoring eosinophil activity in asthma. Arch Dis Child 73: 413–417
37. Wilson R, Cole PJ (1988) The role of bacterial products on ciliary function. Am Rev Respir Dis 138: 549–55
38. Essen-Zandvliet EE van, Hughes MD, Waalkens HJ et al (1993) Effects of 22 months of treatment with inhaled corticosteroids and/or beta-2-agonists on lung function, airway responsiveness, and symptoms in children with asthma. Am Rev Respir Dis 146: 547–51
39. Sanchez I, Koster J, de Powell RE et al (1993) Effect of racemic epinephrine and salbutamol on clinical score and pulmonary mechanics in infants with bronchiolitis. J Pediatrics 122: 145–51
40. Tal A, Golan H, Grauer N et al (1996) Deposition pattern of radiolabeled salbutamol inhaled from a metered-dose inhaler by means of a spacer with mask in young children with airway obstruction. J Pediatr 128: 479–84
41. British Guidelines on Asthma Management (1997) Thorax 52 [Suppl 1]: S 1–S 21
42. Taylor DR, Sears MR, Herbison GP et al (1993) Regular inhaled β agonist in asthma: effects on exacerbations and lung functions. Thorax 48: 134–8
43. Kerrebijn KP, Essen-Zandvliet EEM van, Neijens HJ et al (1987) Effect of long-term treatment with inhaled corticosteroids and β-agonist on the bronchial responsiveness in children with asthma. J Allergy Clin Immunol 79: 653–59
44. Craig VL, Bigos D, Brilli RJ (1996) Efficacy and safety of continuous albuterol nebulization in children with status asthmaticus. Pediatr Emerg Care 12: 1–5
45. O'Byrne PM (1997) Treatment of mild asthma. Lancet 349: 818
46. Browne GJ, Penna AS, Phung X et al (1997) Randomised trial of intravenous salbutamol in early management of acute severe asthma in children. Lancet 349: 310–314
47. Kerem E, Levison H, Schuh S et al (1993) Efficacy of albuterol administered by nebulizer versus spacer device in children with acute asthma. J Pediatr 123: 313–7
48. Jones K (1994) Salmeterol in the management of paediatric asthma. Respir Med 88: 639–43
49. Green CP, Price JF (1992) Prevention of exercise-induced asthma by inhaled salmeterol xinafoate. Arch Dis Child 67: 1014–7
50. Lenney W, Pedersen S, Boner AL et al (1995) Efficacy and safety of salmeterol in childhood asthma. Eur J Pediatr 154: 983–90
51. Russell G, Williams DAJ, Weller P et al (1995) Salmeterol xinafoate in

children on high dose inhaled steroids. Ann Allergy, Asthma & Immunol 75: 423–8
52. Omlor GJ, Quinn LM, Schramm CM (1996) Ontogeny of β-adrenergic desensitization in rabbit tracheal smooth muscle. Pediatr Pulmonol 22: 255–62
53. Cheung D, Timmers MC, Zwinderman AH et al (1992) Long-term effects of a long-lasting β_2-adrenoceptor agonist, salmeterol, on airway hyperresponsiveness in patients with mild asthma. N Engl J Med 327: 1198–203
54. Grove A, Lipworth BJ (1995) Bronchodilator subsensitivity to salbutamol after twice daily salmeterol in asthmatic patients. Lancet 346: 201–6
55. Simons FER, Gerstner TV, Cheang MS (1997) Tolerance to the bronchoprotective effect of salmeterol in adolescents with exercise-induced asthma using concurrent inhaled glucocorticoid treatment. Pediatrics 99: 655–9
56. Noble V, Ruggins NR, Everard MI et al (1992) Inhaled budesonide for chronic wheezing under 18 months of age. Arch Dis Child 67: 285–8

Correspondence: Manfred Götz, MD, Professor of Paediatrics, Head, Department of Paediatric and Adolescent Medicine, Wilhelminenspital, Montleartstrasse 37, A-1171 Vienna.

Discussion

Dr. Kummer: Thank you, Manfred. I missed your last sentence in conclusion, I must apologise. Did you say something offending? I think that was a very important statement. And I would like to have a few questions and comments. Dr. Block?

Dr. Block: It is known to a number of clinicians working in the field with NO, that infants, once they have problems with lung function, will have big benefits from inhalation of NO. Do you know of any evidence or recent information showing that inhalation of NO could stimulate beta receptor function as corticosteroids do?

Dr. Götz: Not in wheezing conditions in that age group. We know of NO for instance in patients with congenital heart disease, but we have no data thus far on the wheezing age group 0–3 years. Cystic fibrosis has been associated with NO, but that is all that is presently available to that question. But I'm sure the future will lead to the appropriate studies.

Dr. Kummer: What about the cholinergic receptors? I remember that ipratropium was quite active in resolution of the vagal tone in children, and it was more active than beta agonists. Could you comment on that?

Dr. Götz: Well, as far as I understand the development of cholinergic receptors parallels more or less that of the adrenergic receptors. Now what this means in clinical practice is even less resolved than the issue of the use of beta-adrenergic substances. The data are really one hundred and eighty degrees in opposition, inasmuch as there is a very small group which has done a lot of studies advocating the use of ipratropium bromide and found good bronchodilatation. These data have fallen into disfavour with most pediatricians and they were not able to reproduce his results. So again, beyond the anatomical demonstration of the presence of receptors, we know relatively little about their functional responsiveness in this early age group. And there are reasonably few people at the moment who will go for a treatment with ipratropium bromide, for instance, to relieve bronchospasms. So I think this is another unresolved issue, perhaps for the next asthma forum.

NN: Professor Götz, can you say something about the present role of long-acting beta agonists in pediatric therapy? What are the indications and at which age would you start?

Dr. Götz: Well, the long-acting beta agents have a limited but definite, assured role in the pediatric wheezing conditions like asthma. Two conditions stick out, I think. The one is the nightly wheezing and cough, and the other one is the prevention of exercise induced bronchospasms. I would point these two out primarily as conditions where long-acting beta agents really have a role proper in the management.

Dr. Kummer: One would probably be curious wether it works in infancy or not.

Dr. Götz: There are no data on infancy, but there are data in preschool and in school children.

Dr. Ulmer: Dr. Götz, you gave us an excellent overview. But the problem for me is to measure lung function in small children.

Dr. Götz: You can see what was measured here normally was using either the squeeze technique or the plethysmograph, we measured the flow max at FRC, that is probably the most sensitive index which can be used for establishing the obstruction in the airways and the relief of that. Kramer has shown also that the TGV measured by the plethysmograph is a very nice index but it is obviously something which is not accessible to the vast majority of patients where the treatment necessity does arise continuously.

Dr. Ulmer: And what is your impression on the clinical side?

Dr. Götz: I wish I'd know. Well, we really go along with the recommendations of either the consensus statement or the UK recommendations. Give it a try, but don't be too disappointed if it doesn't work the way you wish it. You're not doing any harm at all. So we have about 12 to 24 hours before we say it doesn't work. And I think this is a reasonable time to observe a child and to see what it actually does. My impression quite definitely is that these infants need relatively higher doses than you would give in an older child or in an adult. It goes up to even twice of what you would recommend for a grown-up.

Long-acting beta-agonists in exercise induced asthma

*B. Villiger**

Summary

Exercise induced asthma (EIA) is commonly defined as a bronchial obstruction which usually occurs 6 to 8 minutes after starting a submaximal exercise, reaching its maximum 3 to 20 minutes after the end of exercising and disappearing spontaneously after 30 to 120 minutes.

An exercise induced component can be seen in 80–100 % of asthmatic children and in 50–80 % of adult asthmatics.

Our former concept, that EIA is merely a special manifestation of a non-specific bronchial hyperreactivity (BHR) is no longer tenable. Today we have to assume that EIA must depend on other factors which are clearly different from the effect of the test substances (Methacholin, Histamin) usually applied to measure BHR. Martin et al. (1980) were able to demonstrate a clear dissociation between exercise induced and pharmacologically induced bronchial obstruction.

Beta-2 agonists are the most effective agents to prevent EIA, if taken 15 to 20 min. before exercise. The great advantage of formoterol and salmeterol, compared with short acting ones like salbutamol or terbutaline, lies in the marked prolongation of protection against EIA, namely 9 to 12 hours, while the short acting agents, in an equipotent dose, yield a protection of only 2 to 4 hours.

---

* The author apologizes for not being able to furnish a full manuscript.

Cheung (1992) found that inhaled salmeterol resulted in a marked tolerance with a highly significant decrease in protection against methacholin provocation. We tried to challenge these findings by designing a pilot study with 8 elite athletes suffering from moderate EIA for the assessment of long-term protection by salmeterol in an exercise test which was performed 6 hours after inhalation (unpublished data).

After 4 weeks of treatment there was no difference in delta FEV_1 of PEF compared to the initial reaction, so the development of tolerance against salmeterol seemed unlikely in EIA. Nevertheless, it seems justified to add topical steroids to the treatment with long-acting beta-2-agonists to reduce underlying BHR.

In conclusion, long-acting beta-2 agonists are highly superior to the short acting ones in EIA in terms of duration of effect. These findings suggest a particular usefulness in children whose radius of activity and protection from EIA can be favourably influenced over the entire day.

Correspondence: Dr. Beat Villiger, Swiss Olympic Medical Center, Sportmed SO, Grüenistrasse 18, CH-7270 Davos Platz, Switzerland.

Discussion

Dr. Kummer: Thank you, Dr. Villiger. I think this was a very interesting and informative study, because the effect of exercise seems to be quite different in people. Particularly the athletes seem to form a group that might be for one reason or the other different from the average consumer, the average young people or middle-aged people who suffer from exercise induced asthma.

Dr. Selroos: I have two questions. I know that salmeterol has been approved by the International Olympic Committee. What about formoterol? That's my first question.

The second is a technical one. With your experience, how frequently can you perform exercise tests without having one test influencing the response at the second, when you are testing long-acting beta-agonists.

Dr. Villiger: As regards your first question. I think we would have done these studies in 1992, 93, but then because of the problems we had with clenbuterol and the case of Miss Krabbe (German sprint champion), everything was banned. So we stopped again. And now, last October, we finally got through that the International Olympic Committee allowed salbutamol, because it's so close to salmeterol, but formoterol is still banned, and when you use it you are considered doped.

The second thing: We normally use an interval of six hours between tests. It has been shown that by then you are beyond the refractory period. After four hours, at least in lung function, you can't find any blocking by prostaglandins which is characteristic for the refractory period. So I think it's worthwhile to use an interval of six hours.

Dr. Kummer: To my personal understanding, what is the time course? So you say, the athletes get up early in the morning, the competition starts at noon and lasts for, how long?

Dr. Villiger: Two hours. The most will be two and a half hours.

Dr. Kummer: When is then the urine checked? Is it checked afterwards or before they go to the competition?

Dr. Villiger: It's absolutely always after the competition within a few hours, whenever he or she can give a urine sample. You can detect salbutamol in urine nowadays for about thirty-six hours and salmeterol even after five days.

Dr. Kummer: The regular inhaled dose?

Dr. Villiger: Yes.

Dr. Kummer: Miss Krabbe ingested clenbuterol?

Dr. Villiger: Yes, combination tablets with ambroxol.

Dr. Kummer: So this beta-agonist was applied via the systemic route. But I think it's amazing that this minute dose that you inhale shows up in the urine in a concentration that is still detectable.

Dr. Villiger: The half-life in blood is two minutes. And you find it at least five days later, still in the urine. So it's amazing what the people in charge of doping control can do nowadays.

Dr. Kummer: Let me raise another point. There was an intriguing paper in Thorax lately by Grove and Lipworth (1996, 51:54). And they felt that a modulation of the basic sympathetic nervous system level could influence the reaction to formoterol or beta blocking agents. He found that when you increase your sympathetic activity by exercise, and you give formoterol in this situation, it acts like a beta blocker. So I'm not quite sure whether this has any impact on clinical medicine, that somebody inadvertently takes formoterol too late and then gets worse with his EIA. But how do you feel about it?

Dr. Villiger: Well, this seems of more concern for cardiology. There have been basic science studies about that. And as far as I know, there's no clinical relevance to that.

Dr. Anderson: If I may just comment. Unfortunately, formoterol doesn't have any beta-blocking liability at all. I don't know the paper, but pharmacologically formoterol doesn't block the beta-2 receptor at all.

Salmeterol and oral steroid treatment

G. Boyd

Consultant Respiratory Physician,
Stobhill Hospital, Glasgow, Scotland

Summary

Current international guidelines for asthma management recommend the introduction of supportive long acting bronchodilator therapy to be used in conjunction with maximal levels of inhaled corticosteroids, particularly before the introduction of long term oral corticosteroid therapy. A study in severe asthmatics, who were under consideration for the introduction of oral corticosteroid treatment, demonstrated that the addition of Salmeterol to maximal doses of inhaled corticosteroids significantly improved the overall level of asthma control so that in some patients the need to employ long term oral corticosteroid therapy was delayed or prevented.

Salmeterol introduced earlier in milder forms of asthma offers an additional option to increasing the level of inhaled corticosteroid therapy and further more symptom control can be maintained with lower levels of anti-inflammatory medication. The effectiveness of Salmeterol in influencing the level of corticosteroid requirement at different stages of the asthmatic process is a valuable therapeutic asset and promotes a more flexible approach to drug therapy with symptom control achieved with lower levels of anti-inflammatory agent.

Introduction

Current guidelines for the management of asthma embodied internationally in the International Consensus Report on the Diagnosis and Management of Asthma, first published in 1992, [1] established the requirement for the introduction of inhaled corticosteroids in the treatment regime of all but the mildest asthmatics, the dose being adjusted depending on the serverity of the symptoms up to a recommended maximum of 2 mg per day. In the more chronic and severe forms of asthma, the control of symptoms can be difficult to achieve and frequently requires the administration of high levels of both bronchodilator and anti-inflammatory medication. Long term oral corticosteroid therapy may be necessary in the most severe cases in order to secure clinical control. However, although long term oral therapy is effective in achieving this end, it brings with it difficulties associated with significant systemic side effects so that changes in bone metabolism can result in osteoporosis particularly in the elderly, in the post menopausal patients or suppression of the hypothalamic pituitary adrenal axis resulting in low plasma cortisol levels and a reduced response to stress. It becomes a vital clinical consideration, therefore, in the management of chronic asthma to minimise the risk of such drug related side effects. Current management guidelines such as the British Thoracic Society Guidelines published in 1993 [2] and in the further evolution of the thinking in terms of management strategies embodied in the Global Initiatives for Asthma (GINA) published by the National Institutes of Health in January 1995 [3] recommend the introduction of supportive bronchodilator therapy particularly with long acting preparations which should be used in conjunction with maximal levels of inhaled corticosteroids and that this combination should be employed before considering the introduction of long term oral corticosteroid therapy.

The role of long acting inhaled bronchodilator therapy in the form of Salmeterol in the management of asthmatics is still the subject of investigation and detailed evaluation. The initial positioning of this type of therapy was directed towards the more severe forms of asthma although clearly its value is now being confirmed in the management of mild to moderate forms of asthma also. A multi-centred study from the

UK [4] examined the usefulness of adding Salmeterol in a dose of 100 mcg twice daily in patients where long term oral steroid therapy was actively under consideration. 119 chronic symptomatic asthmatics all of whom were receiving at least 1500 mcg daily of inhaled Beclomethasone diproprionate or Budesonide and who were under consideration for maintenance oral corticosteroid therapy were recruited from 15 hospitals within the UK. They were required to have documented history of a minimum of 15 % improvement from baseline in lung function following 400 mcg of inhaled Salbutamol and also of acute exacerbations of asthma on at least 2 occasions in the preceding 18 months. Patients were excluded if they had any concurrent uncontrolled systemic disease, had received treatment for an acute respiratory infection in the preceding 2 weeks or who were unable to demonstrate at least 40 % of their predicted forced expired volume in one second (FEV1) at baseline. After a 2 week baseline period, symptoms, peak flow rates and relief medication were reviewed and only those patients were incorporated into the study who demonstrated at least 2 of the following criteria namely: a night time symptom score which at a minimum reflected symptoms which caused the patients to wake at least once during the night or to waken early, a daytime symptom score with a minimum level of symptoms which were frequent during the day but which did not interfere with the days activities, the use of at least 8 puffs of a relief medication; or a diurnal variation in the peak expiratory flow rate of at least 15 %, on at least 3 of the preceding 7 days. Those who satisfied these criteria were then randomised to receive either Salbutamol 100 mcg twice daily or a matching placebo via a diskhaler delivery system for a 12 week period. Throughout this time they continued to received Salbutamol via a metered dose inhaler for relief of bronchospasm and they continued their usual prophylactic asthma therapy throughout. 97 patients completed the study (47 in the Salmeterol group, and 50 in the placebo group).

The addition of Salmeterol 100 mcg twice daily in this group of individuals on a maximal level of inhaled steroids resulted in 3 observed improvements of importance. Firstly, there was a significant increase ($p = 0.002$) in the increase in proportion of symptom free nights experienced by those receiving Salmeterol (33 %) compared with placebo

(13 %). Secondly, there was a significant decrease ($p = 0.002$) in the daily use of relief medication with a mean decrease of 5.1 doses per day with Salmeterol compared to 2.5 doses per day with the placebo preparation. Thirdly, there was a significant improvement in the morning peak expiratory flow rate achieved after one month in the Salmeterol treated group which persisted throughout the whole treatment period with an estimated treatment difference of 22 litres per minute.

This study, therefore, demonstrated that the introduction of Salmeterol in the treatment regime of chronic asthmatics who were already receiving maximum doses of inhaled corticosteroids had a significant influence on the level of symptoms with an overall improvement in asthma control. Appropriate introduction of Salmeterol, therefore, in some individuals with this level of asthmatic problem could delay or even prevent the requirement for adopting long term oral corticosteroid therapy as the inevitable next step and last resort in treatment. The drug was well tolerated in this group of individuals and the adverse events that were experienced tended to relate more to the severity of the patients existing condition than to the therapeutic agent that was introduced.

It has been shown from the information obtained from 2 major multi-centre investigations [5, 6] that if symptomatic patients who were receiving inhaled corticosteroid routinely were treated with Salmeterol then greater benefit was reported following the introduction of Salmeterol than by doubling the dose of their inhaled corticosteroid therapy. These patients, of course, were not as severe asthmatics as those previously described in that they had no history of exacerbations but their symptoms warranted an adjustment to their therapy to secure better control. In each of these 3 studies the effective outcomes of the treatment regime could be defined within the current Asthma Management Guidelines [2, 3] namely to achieve a reduction in the level of symptoms with the least possible use of relief bronchodilators with demonstrable improvement in pulmonary function and as far as possible a reduction in the limitation of activity all within the constraint of the least possible adverse drug effects. It is clear that Salmeterol satisfies the majority of these criteria and in different grades of asthma severity can offer a further therapeutic option to increasing the level of inhaled corticosteroid therapy. In those patients most severely affected where oral corticosteroid usage is contemplated, Salmeterol appears to offer an effective therapeutic option prior to resorting to systemic corticosteroid usage in those chronic asthmatics who are already receiving high dose inhaled anti-inflammatory medication.

There is now increasing evidence in the literature that the introduction of a long acting inhaled bronchodilator in the form of Salmeterol earlier within the structure of the current guidelines than is at present recommended can influence the level of inhaled corticosteroid anti-inflammatory agent that is required to secure symptom control and permission overall reduction in the amount of inhaled corticosteroid that is required. Preliminary data [7] demonstrated that the introduction of Salmeterol at 50 mcg twice daily in a group of 86 patients on a minimum of 400 mcg of Beclomethasone dipropionate or equivalent drug over a 6 month period reduced the requirement for relief bronchodilator usage, increased the morning and evening peak expiratory flow rate by a mean of 19 and 16 litres per minute respecitvely and also had a significant influence on symptom free days and nights. In addition, it reduced the overall steroid usage from a mean of 677 mcg to 563 mcg ($p < 0.001$) of inhaled corticosteroid. Preliminary data presented recently from Denmark [8] characterised patients' requirement for inhaled steroid therapy and then by using a predefined set of criteria reduced inhaled BDP by 200 mcg per week until asthma controlled could no longer be maintained. The lowest effective dose of inhaled BDP for each individual patient was therefore identified and observed the effect of Salmeterol or placebo on this process. 12 out of 15 patients receiving Salmeterol were able to reduce the level of BDP required for effective control of symptoms by 50% or greater and this steroid reduction was not associated with any changes in the peak expiratory flow rate or measurements of the forced expired volume in one second. It was also noted that Salmeterol treatment was associated with a decrease in symptoms and an increase in days without symptoms. Overall, therefore, further information is now emerging that suggests, certainly in the short term, that the addition of Salmeterol is associated with the reduced need for inhaled steroids in patients who are steroid dependant without any loss of asthma control. Thus the inclusion of Salmeterol not only offers a steroid sparing effect in reducing the requirement to progress to oral corticosteroid therapy in patients receiving high dose inhaled corticosteroid therapy as currently recommended in the management guidelines but also appears to offer significant steroid sparing effects in milder asthmatics who require lower doses of inhaled corticosteroids for symptom control. The place for Salmeterol in the management of severe chronic asthma appears to be established but the challenge of the newer information which is accumulating in terms of steroid sparing effects in the milder forms of asthma must be to stimulate more extensive studies to evaluate its potential in the longer term therapeutic requirements for control of the milder asthmatic. To achieve the satisfactory control of any patient's symptoms and to optimise the effectiveness of asthma control, requires a balance between the use of anti-inflammatory and bronchodilator agents tailored to suit individual requirements. The apparent effectiveness of Salmeterol in influencing the level of corticosteroid requirement at different stages of the asthmatic process is likely to prove a valuable asset in the therapeutic armamentarium for asthma management and will promote a more flexible approach to the balance of drug therapy enabling patients to achieve a more successful level of clinical outcome and a more effective quality of life.

References

1. International consensus report on the diagnosis and management of asthma (1992) Clinical and Experimental Allergy 22 [Suppl]: 1–72
2. British Thoracic Society and others (1993) Guidelines on the management of asthma. Thorax 48 [Suppl]: S 1–S 24
3. Global Initiative for Asthma. Publication No 95-3659, January 1995. National Institutes of Health.
4. G Boyd on behalf of a UK Study Group (1995) Salmeterol xinafoate in asthma patients under consideration for maintenance oral corticosteroid therapy. Eur Respir J 8: 1494–1498
5. Woolcock A, Lundback BO, Ringdal NILS, Jacques LA (1996) Comparison of addition of salmeterol to inhaled steroids with doubling of the dose of inhaled steroids. Am J Crit Care Medicine 153: 1481-8
6. Greening AP, Ind PW, Northfield M, Shaw G on behalf of Allen & Hanburys Limited UK Study Group (1994) Added salmeterol versus higher-

dose corticosteroid in asthma patients with symptoms on existing inhaled corticoster. The Lancet 344: 219–224
7. Tattersfield AE, Wilding P, Thompson-Coon J, Clark M, Lewis S (1996) Efficacy and safety of long term treatment with Salmeterol in Adults with Asthma. Am J Respir Crit Care Medicine 53: A66
8. Pedersen B, Fauischou P, Madsen F, Viskum K, Wilcke T, Dahl R (1996) Salmeterol treatment reduces the need for inhaled steroids in steroid dependent asthmatics – a randomised, double-blind, placebo-controlled parallel group study. Eur Respir 9 [Suppl 23]: 505

Correspondence: Dr. Gavin Boyd, Consultant Respiratory Physician, Stobhill Hospital, 133 Balornock Road, Glasgow G21 3UW, U.K.

Discussion

Dr. Kummer: Thank you, Dr. Boyd, for this very stimulating lecture, because I think and I hope that part of the audience will now be relieved because they treat their patients already in the way that you suggested, and the other part of the audience might be troubled because they might ponder over what we all don't know, namely the late outcome. The relief of the patient within three months is a very advantageous thing but what will be in three years? According to points 6 and 7 of your second slide, is this type of therapy effective in prevention of irreversible airway damage and asthma mortality?

Dr. Selroos: I was surprised to see the improvement in morning peak flow in your placebo group. You didn't mention whether it was necessary to give the patients some courses of oral steroids, but they were candidates for treatment with oral steroids. What happened during the study? How many courses were given, for instance, in the placebo group? And could this improvement in peak flow be a result of that additional treatment?

Secondly, you said that there were statistically significant differences within the group when baseline was compared with treatment. But you didn't say anything about the difference between placebo and the salmeterol group.

Dr. Boyd: The two groups were quite different in terms of their responses. There was a total of 119 absorbed into the study and 97 completed it. Now of those withdrawals, there were 8 or 10 that had clinical exacerbations of their asthma. So in fact, people who required changes in their level of therapy were withdrawn and, as far as possible, within what is really a very heterogeneous group of people, one was trying to concentrate or just observe the effects of salmeterol alone. Where the clinical state varied, they were removed.

I am always suspicious of any data that is shown with big changes in graphs because the eye perceives changes and can make little changes look large, depending on the scale. I think the changes in this group as a whole, when you look at the absolute figures, are really quite small.

In statistical terms, and therefore in group terms, they're important. But I think the critical thing, for me, is that if the patient is more comfortable on this therapy, if the patient is requiring less additional medication and if the patient is not being disturbed at night time, then these clinical elements are much more important than the level of peak flow they actually can achieve. So I'm a little cynical about, let's say, the scientific expression of this type of clinical material. I think it's important that any clinician looks at that with gentle scepticism to make sure that they understand what the true picture is. The basic point is that these patients are better or they are improved, and in clinical terms that is what we pursue as doctors. We then can look for objective proof by coming back to another symposium and listening to the basic scientists telling us why it should be.

Dr. Kummer: Well, we are right down at the aim of this morning's session, namely the philosophy. Should the patient like me more than I like the patient? In terms of what is going to happen in ten years. Will the patient still like me better or like me more, because everything went off smoothly and exactly the way I had planned and wished for the patient to be. If there is no other urgent question or comment, then I would like to have some more discussion on that after Dr. Greening's paper.

Salmeterol and its relationship to treatment with inhaled corticosteroids

A. P. Greening

Consultant Physician, Western General Hospital, Edinburgh, U.K.

Summary

In the context of control of asthma symptoms β_2-agonists have a major role. The long-acting inhaled β_2-agonists, such as salmeterol, would appear to be extremely valuable, not only in control of night-time and exercise related symptoms but also as an addition to inhaled steroids in patients who continue to have symptoms. In this last context the addition of salmeterol is significantly more effective than doubling or more than doubling the dose of inhaled steroid.

Introduction

Earlier presentations have demonstrated the pharmacology and pharmacokinetics of salmeterol. I would now like to review the evidence relating to the clinical activities of the drug, particularly in relationship with the use of inhaled corticosteroids. This, however, has to be placed into more than one context: (a) safety, (b) efficacy, and (c) asthma clinical guidelines. Since 1990 there have been a number of reports suggesting that regular use of short-acting β_2-agonists may lead to worsening control of asthma, increased exacerbations and death [1–3]. The duration of action of salmeterol is such that 12 hourly therapy is the provision of very regular β_2-agonists treatment. I will, therefore, review the potential risks of short-acting β_2-agonists and compare the relevant data for salmeterol. I will then give the evidence for clinical efficacy of salmeterol in clinical situations where long duration of action is particularly pertinent and, finally detail new evidence that suggests the conventional guidelines of asthma management advocating relentless increase in the dose of inhaled corticosteroids may need modification.

Safety aspects of β_2-agonists and salmeterol

Short-acting β_2-agonists

If long-acting β_2-agonists are to be used in the management of asthma one must address the question of safety, in light of the concerns expressed about short-acting β_2-agonists. Several groups of observation need to be considered for adverse potential: rebound bronchoconstriction on cessation of treatment, development of tolerance to their protective effects against bronchoprovocation, potential interaction with the beneficial effects of corticosteroids at the molecular level, and clinical trial or epidemiological data that suggest worsening of the underlying control of asthma with their regular use.

There is evidence that after cessation of short-acting β_2-agonists in asthma there is a rebound decrease in FEV_1 of about 10 % for 1–3 days [4–6], before a return to baseline. A single dose of short-acting β_2-agonist can result in approximately a ten-fold reduction in sensitivity to challenge by histamine or methacholine [7], although this protection is short-lived, lasting for about four hours [8]. However, these acute protective effects appear to decline during regular treatment [9] and after stopping such treatment there is a small rebound increase in bronchial responsiveness [6, 9–11]. Similar effects have been reported for allergen, with both the early [12] and late [13] asthmatic responses appearing to be potentiated after two weeks of regular salbutamol therapy.

A possible association of β-agonist medication and asthma mortality was suggested first in the 1960s [14, 15]. There were conflicting data in support of this observation [16, 17] and the implication made that the association was linked to use of high doses of isoprenaline in particular [18]. Subsequently, case control studies from New Zealand have reported an increased risk of asthma death with one β-agonist, fenoterol, but not another, salbutamol [19–21]. Reviews of the New Zealand asthma mortality epidemic have confirmed the association with fenoterol [22, 23]. An epidemiological study from Canada indicated an increased risk of death or near death from asthma with use of either fenoterol or salbutamol [3]. However, a further analysis of the data has suggested that the risks were probably related to those patients whose asthma was deteriorating and poorly controlled and were, therefore, increasing their use of bronchodilator therapy [24]. This would be consistent with the clinical observation that patients with poorly controlled disease are at greatest risk of death. A meta-analysis of six case-control studies concluded that there was a statistically significant, but extremely small, association between the use of β-agonists and asthma death but that this was limited to the use of drug by nebuliser [25]. There has been less emphasis on morbidity and asthma in association with β-agonist use. Much discussion ensued following the publication by Sears et al. [1] of a crossover study comparing regular and as required fenoterol. Although many of the features of the study design were admirable far fewer patients completed the study than had been calculated for adequate power and the methods of analyses between the two groups are open to criticism.

There can be little doubt that there are effects on lung function and bronchial reactivity associated with regular use of β_2-agonists that may put the patient at potential risk. However, the clinical and epidemiological data do not prove there is an actual, rather than theoretical, clinical risk. They perhaps do highlight what most clinicians believe, namely that patients with poorly controlled asthma are at greater risk and are likely to be using greater amounts of bronchodilator. There remains the question as to whether some β-agonists with greater degrees of β_1 effects, such as isoprenaline and fenoterol, have greater degrees of risk than more β_2-specific drugs. Finally, because the duration of action of the short-acting drugs is so short even absolutely regular six-hourly medication would still give peaks and troughs of effect, and no patient will be that adherent to such a treatment regimen. It is more logical, therefore, to use short-acting β-agonists as required, and use the frequency of such treatment as an indicator of asthma control.

Salmeterol

There is no evidence to suggest that rebound bronchoconstriction occurs after regular use of salmeterol. No study has shown a rebound in bronchial hyperresponsiveness, but there are mixed views as to whether there is a decrease in the degree of protection against a challenge. Cheung and Colleagues found the tenfold reduction in methacholine sensitivity at the beginning of the study reduced to a twofold protection after four weeks of regular therapy with salmeterol [26]. Booth et al., on the other hand, found no reduction in protection over a similar time period [27]. Some of the patients in this study were also taking corticosteroids, and the power of the study was lower. Preliminary data suggest that there may be a loss of protection against allergen challenge with regular use of salmeterol [28]. A loss of protection against exercise challenge has also been reported [29]. This, however, needs confirmation since numbers were small and some patients were omitted from analysis [30].

Long acting inhaled β_2-agonists have only been widely prescribable for a limited period of time, 1990 at the earliest in some countries. Determining their effect on mortality is therefore difficult. In a UK post-marketing surveillance study of salmeterol the use of that long-acting β_2-agonist was not associated statistically with an increased rate of death [31]. One might also obtain an indirect assessment of effect on mortality by looking at the asthma death reates in a large population country after the introduction of a long acting β_2-agonist. Patient exposure to salmeterol amounted to 57000 patient years in the first two years of availability in England and Wales. A fall in asthma mortality occurred in this period, arguing against an increased risk of asthma mortality with use of salmeterol [32]. Morbidity is best assessed in long duration, large number studies, looking at asthma exacerbation rates. While there has not been such a study in patients selected to be at risk of asthma exacerbations the published data thus far are reassuring. In two large twelve-month studies salmeterol was compared with regular salbutamol with the salmeterol patients having fewer exacerbations [33, 34]. The rate of exacerbations tended to decline over the twelve months, which would argue against the long-acting β_2-agonist leading to poorer asthma control. These studies were not placebo controlled but similar results were obtained in two multicentre studies in the USA in which salmeterol was compared with regular and as required salbutamol [35, 36]. In these the salmeterol limbs had the lowest asthma exacerbation rates (1.6 per 1000 patient days). The highest rates occurred in the on demand salbutamol limbs (2.9 per 1000 patient days).

Clinical positioning of salmeterol

The mechanisms of long duration of action of salmeterol have been discussed earlier. Given that the evidence is that regular use of this drug is safe, there are two very obvious clinical circumstances for application and a third that requires us to reconsider asthma management guidelines: nocturnal asthma, exercise-induced asthma, and asthma that is still causing symptoms despite the use of inhaled corticosteroids.

Nocturnal asthma

Salmeterol, in early studies, was effective in controlling nocturnal symptoms [37, 38] and was shown to abolish nocturnal wakening [39]. In that study Douglas' group found no difference between doses of 50 µg or 100 µg twice daily. Salmeterol has also been shown to be more effective in controlling nocturnal asthma than established therapies such as theophylline [40, 41]. We have studied the effect of adding salmeterol to the existing regimen in patients with severe nocturnal asthma despite the use of high dose (mean 1300 µg per day) inhaled corticosteroids [42]. In this placebo controlled study we found salmeterol effective in reducing nocturnal symptoms and awakenings, and the overnight fall in PEF. Again 50 µg appeared as effective as 100 µg, twice daily.

Exercise-induced asthma

Protection against exercise-induced asthma (EIA) for a substantial length of time would be of great benefit particularly to those with random periods of spontaneous exercise, such as schoolchildren, might benefit most. One study looked at the duration of protection offered by salmeterol against EIA in 13 children. All 13 retained complete protection even at 9 hours after dosing [43]. While this and other studies demonstrate efficacy the numbers of subjects are small. However, one recent multicentre study in the USA, has compared placebo with salbutamol 200 µg and salmeterol 50 µg single dose in 161 adolescents and young adults [44]. Complete protection against exercise induced bronchoconstriction was seen in approximately 60 % of salmeterol treated subjects even at 11.5h after dosing (Fig. 1).

Asthma management guidelines

Control of the airways inflammation is deemed to be the central role of asthma management and inhaled corticosteroids are the recommended first line of treatment in national and international guidelines [45, 46]. If control of asthma is not obtained by low doses of inhaled steroids the guidelines advocate higher, and then higher still, doses of inhaled steroids. The exception to this advice has been within the Swedish national guidelines [47]. These have advocated an alternative when moderate doses of inhaled steroids have been reached, such that if a patient remains symptomatic while taking 800 µg per day then either of

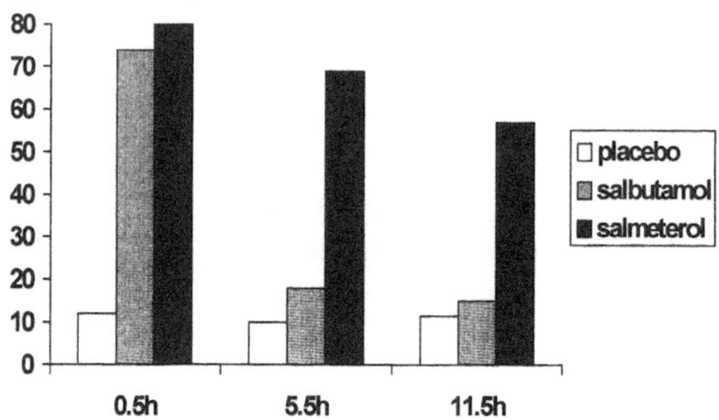

Fig. 1. The percentage of patients showing complete protection against exercise induced asthma at 0.5, 5.5, and 11.5h after dosing with placebo, salbutamol 200 µg and salmeterol 50 µg (From reference [44])

two approaches are recommended: (a) increase the dose of inhaled steroid, or (b) keep the dose of inhaled steroid the same and add in a long acting inhaled β_2-agonist. At the time these guidelines were written there were no published studies to support the latter proposition, although there were data to indicate that the dose-response relationships between inhaled steroids and lung function are not linear [48] and may indeed plateau at surprisingly low doses [49–51]. There are, however, now studies that have addressed the very issue of comparison of increasing the dose of inhaled steroids with the addition, to existing doses, of a long acting inhaled β_2-agonist.

Symptomatic asthma despite the use of inhaled steroids

The first study was in general practice, UK based, and looked at 429 patients with relatively mild asthma, symptomatic while taking 200 μg bd beclomethasone dipropionate (BDP) [52]. The study was of six months duration and compared keeping the dose of BDP the same, at 200 μg bd, but adding salmeterol at 50 μg bd, with more than doubling the dose of BDP to 500 μg bd. The second study was hospital based,

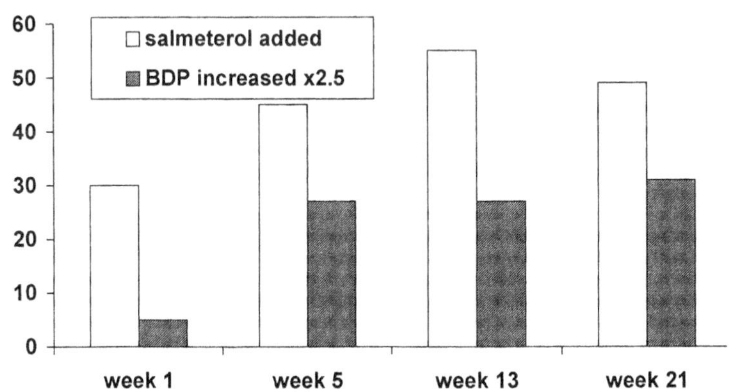

Fig. 2. The percentage decrease in proportion of disturbed nights in patients adding salmeterol 50 μg bd beclomethasone dipropionate (BDP) 200 μg bd and patients increasing their BDP dose to 500 μg bd. The added salmeterol limb was better throughout the six month study (Figure from data in reference [52])

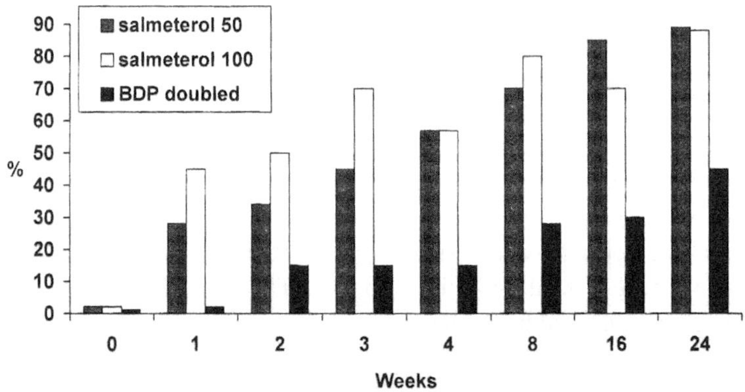

Fig. 3. The percentage of symptom free days in patients adding salmeterol 50 μg bd or 100 μg bd to beclomethasone dipropionate (BDP) 500 μg bd and patients increasing their BDP dose to 1000 μg bd. The added salmeterol limbs were better throughout the six month study, but were not different from each other (Figure from data in reference [53])

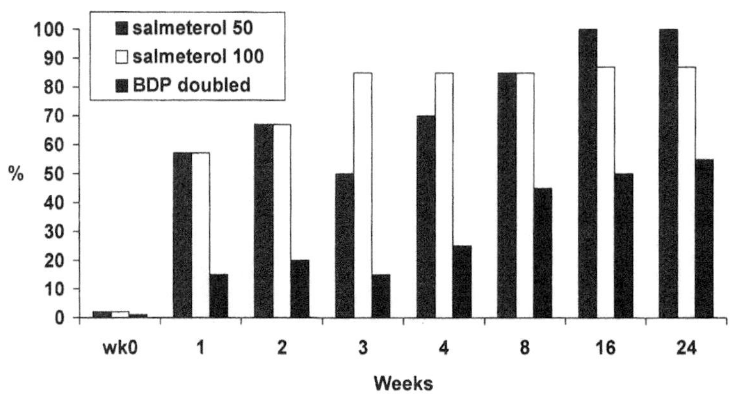

Fig. 4. The percentage of rescue bronchodilator free days in patients adding salmeterol 50 μg bd or 100 μg bd to beclomethasone dipropionate (BDP) 500 μg bd and patients increasing their BDP dose to 1000 μg bd. The added salmeterol limbs were better throughout the six month study, but were not different from each other (Figure from data in reference [53])

international and looked at 738 patients with moderate asthma, symptomatic while taking 500 μg bd BDP [53]. The study was also of six months duration, but had three limbs. In two the dose of BDP was unchanged, at 500 μg bd, with the addition of salmeterol at either 50 μg bd or 100 μg bd, and in the third the dose of BDP was doubled to 1000 μg bd. The two studies were conducted in a double-blind, placebo-controlled, parallel group fashion. Both studies showed that patients achieved better lung function, had fewer daytime or night-time symptoms and used less rescue medication when taking salmeterol in addition to existing doses of inhaled corticosteroids rather than doubling or more than doubling the dose of inhaled steroid (Figs. 2–4). In the international study, with the patients starting at a higher dose of inhaled steroids, the benefits of added salmeterol on symptom control appeared greater than in the milder patients of the UK study, but there was very little additional benefit of using the higher dose of salmeterol. Most importantly the two studies showed no differences between the different limbs with respect to exacerbations of asthma, either number of severity. So, in 1164 patients studied over six months the use of a regular long-acting β-agonist gave no indication of provoking worsening of the underlying asthma, indeed appeared as safe as increasing the dose of inhaled corticosteroids.

In addition a recent study from Tattersfield et al. [54] has suggested that the addition of salmeterol allows a modest dose reduction in inhaled steroid dose, while improving symptom control. They carried out a double-blind, placebo-controlled, cross-over study (6 months per limb) in 101 patients. The dose of inhaled steroid was adjusted throughout the study, in accordance with carefully set criteria. Compared with placebo salmeterol 50 μg bd not only improved morning and evening PEF, gave fewer symptoms and reduced the need for rescue bronchodilator therapy but also allowed a reduction in the daily dose of inhaled steroid (563 μg/day compared with 677 μg/day).

Conclusions

In the context of control of asthma symptoms β_2-agonists have a major role. The long-acting inhaled β_2-agonists, such as salmeterol, would appear to be extremely valuable, not only in control of night-time and exercise related symptoms but also as an addition to inhaled steroids in patients who continue to have symptoms. In this last context the addition of salmeterol is significantly more effective than doubling or more than doubling the dose of inhaled steroid.

References

1. Sears MR, Taylor DR, Print CG, et al (1990) Regular inhaled β-agonist treatment in bronchial asthma. Lancet 336: 1391–6
2. van Schayck CP, Dompeling E, van Herwaarden CLA, et al (1991) Bronchodilator treatment in moderate asthma or chronic bronchitis: continuous or on demand? A randomised controlled study. Brit Med J 303: 1426–31
3. Spitzer WO, Suissa S, Ernst P, et al (1992) The use of β-agonists and the risk of death and near death from asthma. N Engl J Med 326: 501-6
4. Trembath PW, Greenacre JK, Anderson M, et al (1979) Comparison of four week's treatment with fenoterol and terbutaline aerosols in adult asthmatics. A double blind crossover study. J Allergy Clin Immunol 63: 395–400
5. Harvey JE, Tattersfield AE (1982) Airway response to salbutamol: effect of regular salbutamol inhalation in normal, atopic and asthmatic subjects. Thorax 37: 280-7
6. Wahedna I, Wong CS, Wisniewski AFZ, et al (1993) Asthma control during and after cessation of regular $beta_2$-agonist treatment. Am Rev Respir Dis 148: 707–12
7. Bel EH, Zwinderman AH, Timmers MC, et al (1991) The protective effect of a β_2-agonist against excessive airway narrowing in response to bronchoconstrictor stimuli in asthma and chronic obstructive lung disease. Thorax 46: 9–14
8. Gongora HC, Wisniewski AFZ, Tattersfield AE (1991) A single-dose comparison of inhaled albuterol and two formulations of salmeterol on airway activity in asthmatic subjects. Am Rev Respir Dis 144: 626–9
9. Vathenen AS, Knox AJ, Higgins BG, et al (1988) Rebound increase in bronchial responsiveness after treatment with inhaled terbutaline. Lancet i: 544–8
10. Kraan J, Kroeter GH, van der Mark TW, et al (1985) Changes in bronchial hyperreactivity induced by 4 weeks of treatment with anti-asthmatic drugs in patients with allergic asthma: a comparison between budesonide and terbutaline. J Allergy Clin Immunol 76: 628–36
11. Kerrebijn KF, van Essen-Zandvliet EEM, Neijens HJ (1987) Effect of long term treatment with inhaled corticosteroids and β-agonists on the bronchial responsiveness in children with asthma. J Allergy Clin Immunol 79: 653–9

12. Cockroft DW, McPharland CP, Britto SA, et al (1993) Regular inhaled salbutamol and airway responsiveness to allergen. Lancet 342: 833–7
13. Cockroft DW, O'Byrne PM, Swystun VA, et al (1995) Regular use of inhaled albuterol and the allergen-induced late asthmatic response. J Allergy Clin Immunol 96: 44–9
14. Speizer FE, Doll R, Heaf P (1968) Observations on recent increase in mortality from asthma. Br Med J 1: 335–9
15. Speizer FE, Doll R (1968) A century of asthma deaths in young people. Br Med J 3: 245-6
16. Gandevia B (1968) The changing pattern of mortality from asthma in Australia. Med J Aust 1: 747-52 and 884–91
17. Inman WHW, Adelstein AM (1969) Rise and fall of asthma mortality in England and Wales in relation to use of pressurised aerosols. Lancet ii: 279–85
18. Stolley P (1972) Asthma mortality: why the United States was spared an epidemic of deaths due to asthma. Am Rev Respir Dis 105: 883–90
19. Crane J, Pearce N, Flatt A, et al (1989) Prescribed fenoterol and death from asthma in New Zealand, 1981–1983: case control study. Lancet i: 279–85
20. Pearce N, Grainger J, Atkinson M, et al (1990) Case-control study of prescribed fenoterol and death from asthma in New Zealand, 1977–1981. Thorax 45: 170-5
21. Grainger J, Woodman K, Pearce N, et al (1991) Prescribed fenoterol and death from asthma in New Zealand, 1981–1987: a further case control study Thorax 46: 105–11
22. Pearce N, Beasley R, Crane J, et al (1995) End of the New Zealand asthma mortality epidemic. Lancet 345: 41–4
23. Beasley R, Burgess C, Crane J, et al (1995) The New Zealand asthma mortality epidemic. Clin Sci 88: 14–7
24. Suissa S, Blais L, Ernst P (1994) Patterns of increasing β-agonist use and the risk of fatal or near-fatal asthma. Eur Respir J 7: 1602–9
25. Mullen M, Mullen B, Carey M (1993) The association between beta-agonist use and death from asthma. A meta-analytic integration of case-control studies. JAMA 270: 1842–5
26. Cheung D, Timmers MC, Zwinderman AH, et al (1992) The prolonged effects of a long-acting β_2-adrenoceptor agonist, salmeterol, on airway hyperresponsiveness in patients with mild asthma. N Engl J Med 327: 1198–203
27. Booth H, Fishwick K, Harkawat R, et al (1993) Changes in methacholine induced bronchoconstriction with the long acting $beta_2$-agonist salmeterol in mild to moderate asthmatic patients. Thorax 48: 1121–4
28. Giannini D, Carletti A, Dente FL, et al (1995) Tolerance to salmeterol in allergen induced bronchoconstriction. Am J Resp Crit Care Med 151: A39
29. Ramage L, Lipworth BJ, Ingram CG, Cree IA, Dhillon DP (1994) Reduced

protection against exercise induced bronchoconstriction after chronic dosing with salmeterol. Resp Med 88: 363–8
30. Ramage L. Beta$_2$-adrenergic agonists in asthma. MD Thesis, University of Aberdeen, UK (submitted)
31. Castle W, Fuller R, Hull J, et al (1993) The Serevent nationwide surveillance study. Brit Med J 306: 1034–7
32. Devoy MAB, Fuller RW, Palmer JBD (1995) Are there any detrimental effects of the use of inhaled long-acting β_2-agonists in the treatment of asthma. Chest 107: 1116–24
33. Britton MG, Earnshaw JS, Palmer JBD (1992) A twelve month comparison of salmeterol with salbutamol in asthmatic patients. Eur Respir J 5: 1062–7
34. Lundback B, Rawlinson DW, Palmer JBD (1993) Twelve month comparison of salmeterol and salbutamol as dry powder formulations in asthmatic patients. Thorax 48: 148–53
35. Pearlman DS, Chervinsky P, LaForce C, et al (1992) A comparison of salmeterol with albuterol in the treatment of mild to moderate asthma. N Engl J Med 327: 1420–5
36. D'Alonzo GE, Nathan RA, Henochowicz S, et al (1994) Salmeterol xinofoate as maintenance therapy compared with albuterol in patients with asthma. JAMA 271: 1412–6
37. Dahl R, Earnshaw JS, Palmer JB (1991) Salmeterol: a four week study of a long-acting beta-adrenoceptor agonist for the treatment of reversible airways disease. Eur Respir J 4: 1178–84
38. Britton MG, Earnshaw JS, Palmer JB (1992) A twelve month comparison of salmeterol with salbutamol in asthmatic patients. Eur Respir J 5: 1062–67
39. Fitzpatrick MF, MacKay T, Driver H, Douglas NJ (1990) Salmeterol in nocturnal asthma: a double-blind, placebo controlled trial of long-acting inhaled β_2-agonist. Br Med J 301: 1365–68
40. Muir JF, Bertin L, Georges D (1992) Salmeterol versus slow-release theophylline combined with ketotifen in nocturnal asthma: a multicentre trial. Eur Respir J 5: 1197–1200
41. Fjellbirkeland L, Gulsvik A, Palmer JBD (1994) The efficacy and tolerability of inhaled salmeterol and individually dose-titrated, sustained-release theophylline in patients with reversible airways disease. Respir Med 88: 599–607
42. Matusiewicz SP, Dewar M, Howie SEM, Grenning AP (1993) Salmeterol therapy for severe nocturnal asthma does not influence blood lymphocyte and monocyte cell surface activation. Am Rev Respir Dis 147: A980
43. Green CP, Price JF (1992) Prevention of exercise induced asthma by inhaled salmeterol xinofoate. Arch Dis Child 67: 1014–17
44. Kemp JP, Dockhorn RJ, Busse WW, Bleeker ER, van As A (1994) Prolonged effect of inhaled salmeterol against exercise-induced bronchospasm. Am J Resp Crit Care Med 150: 1612–1615

45. International consensus report on the diagnosis and management of asthma (1992) Clin Exp Allergy 22 [Suppl]: 1–72
46. Guidelines on the management of asthma (1993) Thorax 48 [Suppl]: S 1–24
47. Workshop: Pharmacological treatments of bronchial asthma II. (1993) 178–9. Läkemedelsverket, Medical Products Agency, Uppsala, Sweden
48. Toogood JH, Lefcoe NM, Haines DSM, et al (1977) A graded dose assessment of the efficacy of beclomethasone dipropionate aerosol for severe chronic asthma. J Allergy Clin Immunol 59: 298–308
49. Gaddie J, Petrie GR, Reid IW, et al (1973) Aerosol beclomethasone dipropionate: a dose-response study in chronic bronchial asthma. Lancet ii: 280–81
50. Hummel S, Lehtonen L and Study Group (1992) Comparison of oral-steroid sparing by high-dose and low-dose inhaled steroid in maintenance treatment of severe asthma. Lancet 340: 1483–87
51. Sears MR, Taylor DR, Print CG, et al (1992) Increased inhaled bronchodilator vs increased inhaled corticosteroid in the control of moderate asthma. Chest 102: 1709–15
52. Greening AP, Ind PW, Northfield M, et al (1994) Added salmeterol versus higher-dose corticosteroid in asthma patients with symptoms on existing inhaled corticosteroid. Lancet 344: 219–24
53. Woolcock A, Lundback B, Ringdal N, Jacques LA (1996) Comparison of addition of salmeterol to inhaled steroids with doubling of the dose of inhaled steroids. Am J Respir Crit Care Med 153: 1481–88
54. Tattersfield AE, Wilding P, Thompson-Coon J, et al (1996) Efficacy and safety of long term treatment with salmeterol in adults with asthma. Am J Respir Crit Care Med 153: A66

Correspondence: Dr. Andrew Greening, Consultant Physician, Respiratory Medicine Clinic, Western General Hospital, Crewe Road South, Edinburgh EH4 2XU, U. K.

Discussion

Dr. Kummer: Thank you, Dr. Greening! I think it is very important for the clinician to know that statistics are extremely important for a general view on a subject but that they might cover up the individual needs and circumstances of the patient you are actually treating. And that is a very important entrance into the discussion that we will finally have under the guidance of Professor Leo Fabbri.

Dr. Fabbri: Andrew, I enjoyed your presentation, so I know that fifty per cent of my lecture is out. But, could you speculate on this concept:

If the patients of these two groups are unstable under the use of the steroids they are taking, it's possible that they have more airway inflammation than you would expect under treatment with steroids. These have been shown to normalize the pathology, at least the cellular shedding and fibrosis. Now you add on one agent that has been proven not to modify the inflammation. So you do achieve same goals: you reduce symptoms, you improve lung function, but you leave the inflammation there. You nicely showed that there is no excess exacerbations. And there is no evidence that the remaining inflammation is responsible for more asthma deaths. But what are your personal thoughts?

Dr. Greening: That's a very important area to consider. You're suggesting that patients who have inflammation that is under-treated or not resolved might go on to develop fixed airways disease long term. And if we're not treating the inflammation adequately, maybe in ten years' time, we may regret that. I've no answer to that. You have to do a ten-year study to prove it. But, I would make the following reflections:

One is that despite our prejudices, inhaled steroids even in high dose do not necessarily suppress all the airways inflammation. And we've done biopsies in patients with really quite substantial asthma, all on high-dose inhaled steroids, and there are a number on systemic steroids as well, they have as many eosinophils in their bronchial biopsies as the untreated mild asthmatic might appear to have. So there are people who do not suppress their airways inflammation even when you give them very high doses of inhaled steroid. And I think that we actually underestimate that. I think we believe that inhaled steroids really do attenuate the inflammation and I think they do for many people. But I believe that some are more severe and persistent asthmatics, that by steroids they are not getting rid of it, and even if you push the dose up very high, you may still find the result disappointing. So that's difficult. You're now saying that you actually need other therapies that might modify the inflammatory base. So I would share your concerns that we might be under-treating the level of inflammation if we simply aim at clinical control of symptoms, and I would certainly be very concerned if doctors were treating their patients with effective symptom relievers and not treating the underlying inflammation at all. And I think it is a concern, maybe in the United States, that people are talking in terms of monotherapy for long-acting inhaled beta-2 agonists. I would be very worried about that. And I display my training and prejudice that I would like to see at least 800 g of inhaled steroid there for people who have persistent asthma. After that you may well have a range of choices of drugs to use.

Dr. Kummer: Thank you. I think the issue is: Are there patients (and apparently there are) who are not improving their inflammation even by increasing from fairly high doses to a tremendous dose of inhaled steroids. But on the other hand, it appears to me that there must be a lot of patients who are very well controlled in terms of their inflammation on a quite low dose of inhaled steroids. And these are the ones in whom the clinician is probably totally justified in adding the long-acting beta agonists rendering the patients asymptomatic.

Dr. Greening: I think there are a lot of those people but I suspect that I don't ever see any of them. They don't get referred to hospital, they'll be so well controlled in general practice.

Dr. Selroos: I think that the effect of inhaled steroids on the inflammatory process is very much dependent on when you start that treatment. I agree that if a patient has had airway inflammation and asthma for ten years, and we start with whatever dose, it's very unlikely that we will see a complete normalisation of the airway mucosa. That has been very nicely shown by Haahtela et al. in their studies.
In Finland our national asthma management guidelines recommend to start treatment of asthma as soon as possible after diagnosis with a high dose of an inhaled steroid, irrespective of asthma severity. With this approach we have seen that asthma control is achieved quite rapidly and that it is possible to gradually reduce the dose of the inhaled steroid with maintained asthma control. Secondly, it is also possible to discontinue the treatment for long periods of time without deterioration of asthma. This probably indicates that the inflammatory lesions have been affected by the early high-dose treatment.

Dr. Greening: That's a very important point. And I think in terms of clinical practice, the guidelines aren't quite too helpful when they talk of steps. You're better thinking of a level that you come in at and start high and come down, is quite a good idea. I'm aware of your data and they are very interesting. There may just be a difference between children and adults. And there's no doubt that in a number of children over a period of time their asthma will appear to go away. I mean, if you look at the incidence, the frequency of asthma is about three times in children than it is in adults. Therefore, a number of children have to lose their asthma. It may be different when you look at adults in terms of whether they actually ever get rid of their airways inflammation or not.

Dr. Selroos: Right. However, I'm not referring to children. We have data in adult patients showing that early treatment with a high dose is clinically very effective. Biopsies also show that in many cases the inflammatory changes disappear as a result of the treatment. However, we do not have follow-up data for sufficiently long periods of time in order to know what happens long term to these patients.

Dr. Ulmer: I think you told us that when you give beta-2 sympathicomimetics on a regular basis, this saves glucocorticosteroids. The question for me is, is this part of a real anti-inflammatory effect or is this only because you open the airways? Keeping open the airways means that you increase clearing mechanism.

Dr. Boyd: If you have the balance of therapy in the patient, then you will optimise the response. I think all the information suggests that there are some people who respond better to inhaled steroids in clinical terms and others respond better to the long-acting reliever preparations. So that the dilemma is: which one fits?

Dr. Boyd: Well, I think this depends on the individual patient.

Dr. Boyd: The biggest problem I have, and the reason why I can only agree in part with what Professor Fabbri has said in that: Hippocrates wrote that the patient stops taking the medicine and gets sick he then blames the doctor. I believe that there are a large number of patients, maybe not your patients, but certainly some of mine, who, when the symptoms go away, the medicine goes away as well. And so we really don't know whether we're protecting them by offering large doses of medication or whether it is the natural history of the condition that produces a different picture. When we consider the step down in treatment as advanced by guidelines, the patient is actually doing that all the time. And we have to be aware of it.

Dr. Ulmer: This is a little different from our experience. We have this special asthma in coal miners, which never goes away. These people need continuous treatment. And we have experiences over 20 years with this group of many hundreds of patients. And we treat them on a regular basis with beta-2 sympathicomimetics and inhaled steroids. And they do extremely well. The life expectancy has increased tremendously since we started with this regular treatment.

Dr. Greening: I think coal miners are a very special case, aren't they?

Dr. Ulmer: Yes, not every obstruction is the same as the other.

Dr. Greening: Maybe the mechanism of induction of hyperreactivity and inflammation is quite different in these patients. I don't know. We've solved the problem in Scotland, we've closed the mines.

Long term treatment with formoterol

M. Rudolf

Consultant Physician, Ealing Hospital, London, U. K., Hon. Senior Lecturer, University London

Summary

The important beneficial characteristics of formoterol can be summarised as follows:

- 12 μg dose has speed of onset within 1–3 minutes and provides bronchodilatation for up to 12 hours
- effective in nocturnal and exercise-induced asthma
- 12 μg twice daily is effective and safe in treatment of patients with reversible airways obstruction
- remains equally effective and safe after one year of continuous treatment
- tolerability profile similar to short-acting $beta_2$-agonists
- no rebound increase in bronchial responsiveness after withdrawal of treatment

Regular treatment with formoterol 12 μg b.i.d. is therefore clearly indicated in moderate-to-severe asthma where patients are not well controlled on regular inhaled steroids and as-needed short-acting inhaled $beta_2$-agonists. Whether or not formoterol should be used in patients with milder disease instead of increasing a low dose of inhaled steroid (as has been suggested by two recent studies with salmeterol [20, 21] remains debatable. However, for those patients who are having problems with inhaled steroids, or for whom nocturnal or exercise-induced symptoms persist despite otherwise good control, formoterol is certainly a reasonable alternative. These recommandations for the use of formoterol are fully in keeping with the indications for long-acting inhaled beta$_2$-agonists suggested by the latest British guidelines on asthma management [22].

Introduction

Short-acting inhaled beta$_2$-agonists provide rapid relief of asthmatic symptoms and have undoubtedly revolutionised the treatment of asthma over the past 25 years. Although there have been some concerns about their safety in recent years, with some questions raised about their possible role in asthma deaths, they nevertheless remain the cornerstone of symptomatic therapy in asthma and they are the medication of choice for the treatment of acute exacerbations of asthma and for the pre-treatment of exercise-induced asthma [1].

The major disadvantage of these drugs is their comparatively short duration of action, with most of the short-acting inhaled beta$_2$-agonists only providing bronchodilatation for upto 4–6 hours. The long-acting inhaled beta$_2$-agonists formoterol and salmeterol have a duration of action lasting more than 12 hours, and therefore offer a number of potential therapeutic advantages. Current International guidelines for asthma management [1] state that "although the position of long-acting inhaled beta$_2$-agonists in asthma therapy has not been clearly defined and further clinical trials are necessary, clinical studies have indicated that chronic treatment with long-acting inhaled beta$_2$-agonists improves symptom scores, decreases nocturnal asthma, improves lung function and decreases the need for rescue use of short-acting inhaled beta$_2$-agonists".

These guidelines go on to state that "long-acting inhaled beta$_2$-agonists may be considered when standard introductory doses of inhaled corticosteroids fail to achieve control of asthma, especially nocturnal symptoms ... but some asthma specialists prefer to add long-acting inhaled beta$_2$-agonists only after a trial of higher doses of corticosteroids continues to reveal symptoms or a need for short-acting inhaled

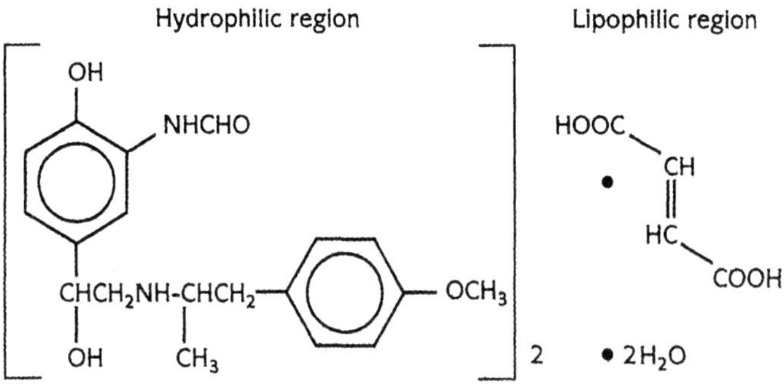

Fig. 1. Chemical formula of formoterol fumarate, showing the hydrophilic region (left) and the lipophilic region (right)

beta$_2$-agonists three to four times a day or more", and that "long-acting inhaled beta$_2$-agonists may also be used to prevent exercise-induced asthma and may provide longer protection than the short-acting beta$_2$-agonists".

This article reviews the clinical trial data of formoterol, with particular emphasis on long term studies, and concludes with specific recommendations for its use in clinical practice.

Clinical pharmacology: onset and duration of action

Formoterol fumarate (Fig. 1) is a highly potent, long-acting, selective beta$_2$ agonist, initially developed as an inhaled bronchodilator in an aerosol metered dose inhaler for use by patients with reversible airways obstruction. It is also available in a dry powder formulation containing micronised drug and lactose, to be inhaled through a dry powder inhaler.

Table 1. Benefits of inhaled formoterol

Effective bronchodilatation in patients with reversible airways obstruction
Rapid onset of action
Long duration of action
Effective in preventing induced bronchoconstriction
No clinical evidence of tolerance in long term use
Effective in twice daily dosage regimen
Low incidence of unwanted effects in adults, children and the elderly

Formoterol has been shown to be both effective and well tolerated in over 100 clinical trials, and its major benefits are summarised in Table 1.

Although, like salmeterol, it is a lipophilic molecule, the mechanism whereby it achieves its long duration of action is different [2]. Detailed biophysical analysis suggests that, following inhalation, some of the drug gain rapid access to the beta$_2$-adrenoceptor (thereby producing fast onset of bronchodilatation) whilst the rest enters the cell membrane phospholipid where it forms a "micro depot" from which it gradually leaches out and is thus available over a prolonged period to stimulate the beta$_2$-adrenergic receptor site [3].

It thus has a faster onset of action that that of salmeterol, and, in experimental comparisons in pharmacological and biophysical tests, formoterol has a relatively high efficacy comparable to the full agonist isoprenaline, whereas salmeterol behaves as a rather weak partial agonist causing less than maximal relaxation of bronchial muscle [4].

Three studies [5, 6, 7] have examined the effect of formoterol at doses of 12 μg and 24 μg, compared with salbutamol dry powder 400 μg and placebo, on the onset of bronchodilatation as measured by changes in specific airways resistance. The results, summarised in Table 2, show the following:

Table 2. Speed of onset

		Improvement in specific airways resistance (%)				
		Study 1 (*n* = 16)		*Study 2* (*n* = 15)		*Study 3* (*n* = 18)
Treatment	***Comparator***	1 min	3 min	1 min	3 min	3 min
Formoterol 24 μg	Placebo	22*	38**	28**	45**	46**
Formoterol 12 μg	Placebo	18	29**	24**	42**	30*
Salbutamol 400 μg	Placebo	18*	37**	31**	38**	–
Formoterol 24 μg	Salbutamol 400 μg	4	1	–3	11	–
Formoterol 12 μg	Salbutamol 400 μg	–1	–12	–10	6	–
Formoterol 24 μg	Formoterol 12 μg	5	12	6	6	22

Onset of bronchodilatation, as measured by percentage improvement in specific airways resistance: single doses of formoterol 12 and 24 μg and salbutamol 400 μg compared to placebo in three studies [5, 6, 7] in patients with stable asthma. * $p < 0.05$; ** $p < 0.01$

- speed of onset within 1–3 minutes of inhalation
- equivalent speed of onset to salbutamol
- no difference between the 12 and 24 μg doses

Four studies [5, 6, 7, 8] in 86 patients have all confirmed the long duration of action of formoterol dry powder at doses of 12 and 24 μg, with statistically and clinically significant changes being observed 12 hours post dosing compared with placebo and salbutamol. The results of one such study [6] in 15 patients are shown in Fig. 2.

Prolonged bronchoprotection, as opposed to bronchodilatation, has been demonstrated in another study [9], specifically designed to examine the extent and duration of protection against exercise-induced bronchoconstriction in 16 patients. In this study, formoterol 12 μg, but not salbutamol 400 μg or placebo, provided protection against exercise challenge at 10 hours after drug inhalation.

Long term efficacy

Most of the clinically relevant data on the long term efficacy and tolerability of formoterol dry powder comes from four large, multicentre

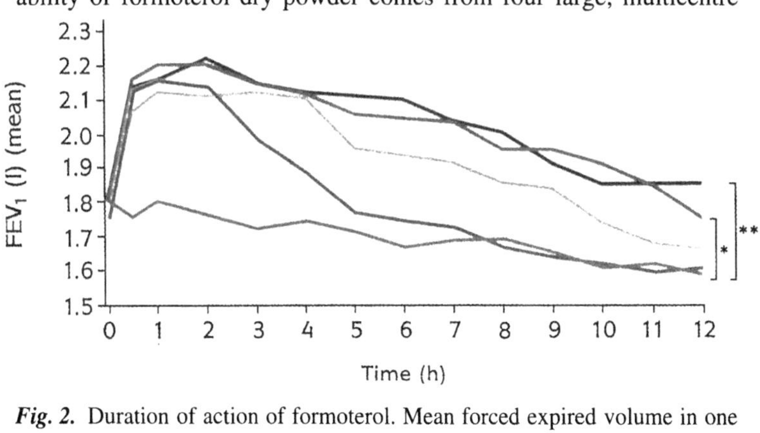

Fig. 2. Duration of action of formoterol. Mean forced expired volume in one second (FEV_1) values during the 12 hours after inhalation of single doses of formoterol 6 μg ——, 12 μg —, and 24 μg —, salbutamol 400 μg —, or placebo —, in 15 patients with stable asthma.

* $p < 0.005$, ** $p < 0.0001$. Increases in FEV_1 at 30 minutes, 1 hour and 2 hours did not differ significantly between the active drugs. (Redrawn from Reference [6])

studies [10, 11, 12, 13] involving 1326 patients with reversible obstructive airways disease. All four of these studies had the same general format: after a run-in period of 1–2 weeks, during which they received either salbutamol 400 μg four times daily or placebo, patients (age range 18–82 years) received either formoterol 12 μg twice daily, formoterol 24 μg twice daily, salbutamol 400 μg four times daily, or placebo in a randomised, double-blind, parallel group design for a period of three months. Clinical assessments were undertaken at the start of the run-inperiod, at baseline, and at four, eight and twelve weeks. In addition, patients recorded their morning and evening peak expriatory flow (PEF), asthma symptom scores both during the day and at night, and their use of salbutamol as rescue medication.

The main primary variable evaluated in all these trials was the pre-dose morning PEF during the week prior to each clinic visit, as specified above. Other variables analysed included spirometric readings at every clinic visit, evening and post-dose PEFs, day- and night-time asthma symptom scores, sleep disturbance scores, need for rescue medication, and overall assessment of efficacy. Tolerability was assessed by haematological and biochemical parameters, pulse rate, blood pressure, electrocardiogram, and adverse event recording. In three of the studies [10, 11, 12], many patients continued with formoterol for a further twelve months in an open design.

Mean pre-dose morning PEFs from one of the studies [11] are shown in Fig. 3, both for the three month comparative trial and for the one year open follow up. Over the first three months, both formoterol 12 and 24 μg twice daily were significantly better than salbutamol, with little to choose between the two doses of formoterol. An overall meta-analysis of mean morning pre-medicatin PEFs in all four studies has confirmed the superiority of formoterol 12 μg b.i.d. over salbutamol q.i.d., with only small insignificant differences between the two doses of formoterol. In all four studies, both doses of formoterol were also superior to salbutamol and placebo on all other variables measured (spirometry at clinic visits, evening and post-dose PEFs, day- and night-time symptom scores, sleep disturbance scores, need for rescue medication with salbutamol), with the single exception of the study [12] on more elderly patients (age range 64–82 years), where staistically significant improve-

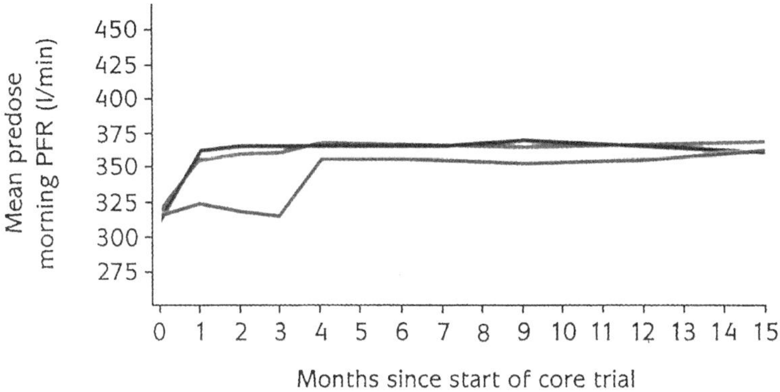

Fig. 3. Peak expiratory flow in one year study. Mean predose morning PEF for patients on formoterol 12 μg twice daily —— for initial 3 months (core trial period) and 1 year follow up; patients on formoterol 24 μg twice daily — for initial 3 months and then formoterol 12 μg twice daily for 1 year follow up; and patients on salbutamol 400 μg four times daily — for initial 3 months and then formoterol 12 μg twice daily for 1 year follow up. Patients who needed to increase their dose of formoterol from 12 μg twice daily to 24 μg twice daily are excluded. (Redrawn from Reference [11])

ments in day- and night-time symptom scores were not observed. This was explained by the finding of much lower symptom scores in this study, presumably due to the known poor perception of symptoms in older patients.

In addition to the improvements in nocturnal symptom scores referred to above, analysis of the numbers of patients who experienced no night-time symptoms at all demonstrated clear superiority for both doses of formoterol (Fig. 4). Two further trials [14, 15], looking specifically at nocturnal asthma in a total of 98 patients, have confirmed that formoterol 12 μg twice daily is effective in decreasing night-time symptoms, nocturnal wheezing, and the amount of sleep disturbance.

As mentioned earlier, three of the long-term studies [10, 11, 12] continued as open, non-comparative extensions for up to one year. Irrespective of trial medication during the initial three month phase, patients continued on formoterol 12 μg twice daily, although they could increase the dose to 24 μg twice daily if necessary; formoterol 12 μg was used

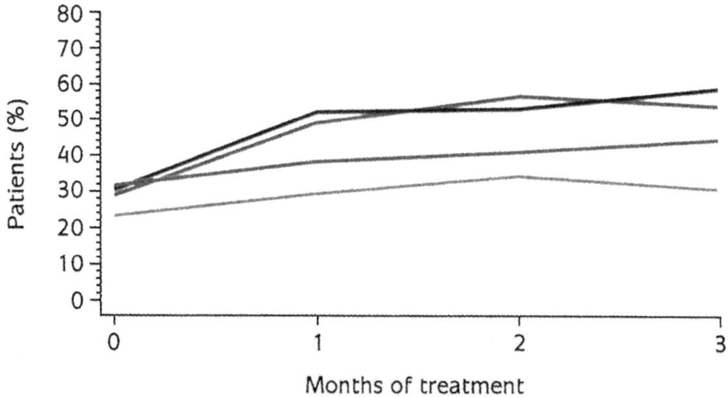

Fig. 4. Nocturnal symptoms in three month studies. Percentage of patients who experienced no night-time asthma symptoms in the week prior to each clinic visit, based on treatment received
— formoterol 12 µg twice daily
— formoterol 24 µg twice daily
— salbutamol 400 µg four times daily
— placebo

as rescue medication, up to a maximum daily dose of 72 µg. Although the primary purpose of this one year extension was to assess long-term tolerability, efficacy data were also collected.

In general, all the benefits noted in the three month studies were maintained, and there was no unexpected increase in adverse events with long term use over one year. In particular, as illustrated in Fig. 3, the improvements in PEF obtained during the initial three month phase were sustained for the ensuing year, with no loss of bronchodilator efficacy. In addition, when used as rescue medication, formoterol was found to be both effective and well tolerated, although the need for rescue use was very small (mean 2.8 doses per week, median 0).

Tolerability and safety

Effects of single doses of formoterol up to 96 µg on the cardio-vascular system (heart rate, blood pressure and ECG), and on glucose and potassium levels, have been investigated in a double-blind, placebo-

Table 3. Adverse events. Beta$_2$-agonist-related adverse events by total daily dose in all multiple-dose trials with formoterol dry powder

	Formoterol				Salbutamol		Placebo	
	12 μg b.i.d.		24 μg b.i.d.		400 μg q.i.d.			
	n	%	n	%	n	%	n	%
Total number of patients	727	(100)	302	(100)	370	(100)	137	(100)
Headache	33	(5)	11	(4)	20	(5)	10	(7)
Tremor	11	(2)	12	(4)	8	(2)	1	(< 1)
Dizziness	11	(2)	6	(2)	4	(1)	0	
Agitation	4	(< 1)	0		1	(< 1)	0	
Palpitations	7	(1)	7	(2)	12	(3)	1	(< 1)
Muscle cramps	4	(< 1)	6	(2)	3	(< 1)	0	

controlled, cross-over study [16]. Although small, clinically insignificant dose-dependent effects are seen on all variables, the only potentially relevant clinical effect is a fall in plasma potassium after the 96 μg single dose. Thus the usually recommended dose of 12 μg twice daily allows a more than satisfactory safety margin, even if extra 12 μg doses are taken. Furthermore, as with all the non-pulmonary systemic effects of beta$_2$-agonists, tolerance occurs to hypokalaemia with chronic dosing [17].

Analysis of all adverse events reported from all the multiple dose trials of formoterol dry powder at doses of 12 or 24 μg twice daily reveals nothing that would not be expected with any beta$_2$-agonist (Table 3). The safety profile of formoterol does not appear to be influenced significantly by factors such as age, sex, concomitant medication, or duration of exposure; dose influences the pharmacologically predictable effects of tremor, palpitations and muscle cramps.

Bronchial hyper-responsiveness and tolerance to bronchodilator and bronchoprotective effects

Concern has been expressed that regular beta$_2$-agonist therapy (with either long- or short-acting preparations) may lead to a rebound increase in bronchial responsiveness, and a consequent reduction in bronchoprotective effect, on discontinuation of treatment.

One double-blind, randomised, crossover study [18] specifically designed to address this issue showed that treatment with formoterol 24 µg twice daily in young people (n = 17, mean age 26.3 + 1.4 years) with mild asthma, none of whom were receiving inhaled steroids, was not followed by any rebound increase in bronchial responsiveness after cessation of two week's treatment. There was evidence that a degree of tolerance had occurred to the bronchoprotective effect of formoterol against methacholine challenge, but it is debatable whether or not this was of any clinical relevance.

In a recent double-blind, parallel group clinical trial [19] in 271 patients with asthma, randomised to six months' therapy with either formoterol 12 µg twice daily, salbutamol 200 µg four times daily, or salbutamol on demand, no clinically or statistically significant evidence of development of tolerance to the bronchodilator and bronchoprotective effects of formoterol was observed.

Despite long term clinical trials with formoterol not revealing any evidence of tolerance to its bronchodilator effect, it has nevertheless still been postulated that prolonged receptor occupancy with a long-acting $beta_2$-agonist might lead to receptor down-regulation and the development of subsensitivity. In a placebo-controlled study [17] where 16 asthmatics were treated with formoterol 24 µg b.i.d., analysis of dose response curves to formoterol after four weeks' continuous treatment did not show any significant changes in peak absolute values of FEV_1 or FEF_{25-75}. However, an analysis of the individual changes from baseline did reveal some bronchodilator subsensitivity in terms of both peak and duration of response to cumulative repeated doses of formoterol. Despite this, clinically significant improvements in FEV_1 were still observed after four weeks' treatment with formoterol, PEFs were increased and the need for rescue medication decreased.

Thus, although these two studies [17, 18] have provided evidence of some pharmacological tolerance to formoterol's bronchodilator and bronchoprotective effects, the wealth of clinical data from long term trials suggests that these findings are probably not of any major clinical significance.

Conclusions

The important beneficial characteristics of formoterol can be summarised as follows:

- 12 μg dose has speed of onset within 1–3 minutes and provides bronchodilatation for up to 12 hours
- effective in nocturnal and exercise-induced asthma
- 12 μg twice daily is effective and safe in treatment of patients with reversible airways obstruction
- remains equally effective and safe after one year of continuous treatment
- tolerability profile similar to short-acting $beta_2$-agonists
- no rebound increase in bronchial responsiveness after withdrawal of treatment

Regular treatment with formoterol 12 μg b.i.d. is therefore clearly indicated in moderate-to-severe asthma where patients are not well controlled on regular inhaled steroids and as-needed short-acting inhaled $beta_2$-agonists. Whether or not formoterol should be used in patients with milder disease instead of increasing a low dose of inhaled steroid (as has been suggested by two recent studies with salmeterol [20, 21] remains debatable. However, for those patients who are having problems with inhaled steroids, or for whom nocturnal or exercise-induced symptoms persist despite otherwise good control, formoterol is certainly a reasonable alternative. These recommendations for the use of formoterol are fully in keeping with the indications for long-acting inhaled $beta_2$-agonists suggested by the latest British guidelines on asthma management [22].

Formoterol is not recommended, and indeed in many countries does not have a product licence, for use as rescue bronchodilatation, for which short-acting inhaled $beta_2$-agonists remain the drugs of choice. Nevertheless, patients can be reassured that it is both effective and safe if they have used it in this way. However, repeated use of formoterol (or any other bronchodilator) for rescue indicates inadequate asthma control and other increases in therapy should be considered.

Finally, current evidence indicates that formoterol has no clinically relevant anti-inflammatory effects, and appropriate doses of suitable anti-inflammatory drugs should always be co-prescribed for patients with asthma.

References

1. Global Initiative for Asthma (1995) Global strategy for asthma management and prevention. NHLBI/WHO Workshop report. National Institutes of Health, Publication 95-3659
2. Nelson HS (1995) Beta-adrenergic bronchodilators N Engl J Med 333: 499–506
3. Anderson GP (1993) Formoterol: pharmacology, molecular basis of agonism, and mechanism of long duration of a highly potent and selective $beta_2$-adrenoceptor agonist bronchodilator. Life Sciences 52: 2145–60
4. Anderson GP (1993) Long-acting inhaled beta-adrenoceptor agonists; the comparative pharmacology of formoterol and salmeterol. New drugs in allergy and asthma 1993. Birkhäuser, Basel, pp 253–269
5. Clinical trial report DP/ON2. Data on file, Ciba
6. Wallin A, Sandström T, Rosenhall L, Melander B (1993) Time course and duration of bronchodilatation with formoterol dry powder in patients with stable asthma. Thorax 48: 611–614
7. Clinical trial report DP/DF4. Data on file, Ciba
8. Hendrick DJ, Brambilla R, Bromly CG (1995) Inhaled formoterol dry powder: duration of bronchodilator action following single dose. Eur Respir J 8 [Suppl 19]: 260s
9. Guerin JC, Germain M, Febvre N, Mairon N, Meyer F (1993) Protective effect of formoterol on exercise induced bronchoconstriction 10 hours after inhalation. Eur Respir J 6 [Suppl 7]: 201s
10. Steffensen I, Faurschou P, Riska H et al (1995) Inhaled formoterol dry powder in the treatment of patients with reversible obstuctive airways disease. Allergy 50: 657–663
11. Maesen FPV (1995) Eformoterol versus salbutamol in patients with R.O.A.D. Br J Clin Pract (1995) [Suppl] 81: 8–10
12. Angus RM, Thomson NC (1995) Comparison of the efficacy and tolerability of eformoterol and salbutamol dry powder capsules for inhalation in elderly asthmatic patients. Thorax 50: 469P–470P
13. Clinical trial report DP/RD4 (part of MT/A03). Data on file, Ciba
14. Clauzel A, Lacoste J, Godard P et al (1994) Effect of formoterol powder on nocturnal wheezes. Eur Respir J 7 [Suppl 19]: 238s
15. Clincal trial report DP/NA1. Data on file, Ciba
16. Burgess C, Ayson M, Rajasingham S et al (1994) The cardiovascular and metabolic effects of increasing doses of formoterol in patients with asthma. Eur Respir J 7 [Suppl 18]: 204s

17. Newnham D, Grove A, McDevitt D et al (1995) Subsensitivity of bronchodilator and systemic $beta_2$ adrenoceptor responses after regular twice daily treatment with eformoterol dry powder in asthmatic patients. Thorax 50: 497–504
18. Yates DH, Sussman HS, Shaw MJ et al (1995) Regular formoterol treatment in mild asthma: effect on bronchial responsiveness during and after treatment. Am J Respir and Crit Care Med 152: 1170–74
19. Clinical trial report DP/OD1. Data on file, Ciba
20. Woolcock A, Lundback B, Ringdal OLN et al (1994) Comparison of the effect of addition of salmeterol with doubling the inhaled steroid dose in asthmatic patients. Am J Respir Dis 149: A280
21. Greening AP, Ind PW, Northfield M et al (1994) Added salmeterol versus higher-dose corticosteroid in asthma patients with symptoms on existing inhaled corticosteroids. Lancet 344: 219–224
22. British Thoracic Society (1997) The British guidelines on asthma management. Thorax 52 [Suppl 1]: S 1–S 20

Correspondence: Dr. Michael Rudolf, Department of Respiratory Medicine, Ealing Hospital, Uxbridge Road, Southall Middlesex UB1 3HW, U.K.

Discussion

Dr. Fabbri: Thank you, Dr. Rudolf. The presentation is open for discussion. Andrew? Be provocative, please.

Dr. Greening: I should like to comment on the Lipworth study that you referred to about possible tolerance occurring to the bronchodilator effect of formoterol (Ref. No. 17 of Rudolf's paper). I think one has to address the way in which the data were presented in the original published paper, where it may well be misleading to conclude that there is tolerance to the bronchodilator effect by comparing only the changes in FEV_1 from baseline, i.e. delta FEV_1. The way in which you presented the data, showing the absolute values of FEV_1 and not just the delta FEV_1 is how it should be viewed. I think I am reassured that there is no development of receptor down-regulation.

Dr. Rudolf: I totally agree with you. It is interesting that the absolute FEV_1 data were not given in the original paper and that only the delta values were published. But the absolute values are very reassuring. At the end of the day, whether or not there is some small effect, and on balance I agree that there probably isn't, I honestly can think of no way in which it is of any clinical relevance when you look at all of the other long-term clinical trial data.

Dr. Greening: I agree, and it is a great shame that the absolute FEV_1 data were not published. I was delighted to see all the very clear data you have shown us on formoterol. My only concern is the possible suggestion that formoterol might be used as rescue therapy. Although I wholeheartedly agree with the way you positioned formoterol at the end of your presentation, I think that you cannot say that there is absolute proof of safety if the drug is used for rescue. This is because in the one year follow up data that you presented where formoterol was indeed used for rescue, you said that very few of the patients actually had to use formoterol with any great frequency. To be absolutely certain about safety, you would have to take a group of patients who have multiple exacerbations and treat them prospectively with formoterol as a rescue bronchodilator. There is a good consistency of opinion that long-acting inhaled beta2-agonists should be used only as regular twice daily maintenance bronchodilator therapy and that they should not be used as rescue medication.

Dr. Rudolf: I would agree with that. I specifically said I do not think this drug should be recommended as rescue medication. But we're still faced with the fact that patients don't do what we tell them. And from what data there is, if a patient comes and says, "Oh, I had two extra puffs of formoterol yesterday", I can confidently reassure that patient that this was indeed a safe thing to have done, even though I do not wish him to carry on doing it.

Dr. Anderson: This is really just to educate myself and gain experience from people who've used these drugs in clinical situations in comparison to short-acting drugs. What are the expectations of a rescue medication? What do patients want from rescue and what do clinicians want, what does rescue mean clinically?

Dr. Boyd: Clinically, if any patient on any treatment suddenly feels wheezy, short of breath and tight, he wants to feel better as quickly as possible and he will use a short-acting inhaled beta agonist. It is entirely similar to taking a nitrate when you get angina. You are looking for immediate symptom relief.

Dr. Anderson: And are there any good studies to understand how long an episode lasts for a patient who requires rescue medication and how long is the constriction lasting?

Dr. Boyd: It varies an awful lot from patient to patient. And I think one of the best measures we have of the efficacy of thc long-acting beta-agonists is the decreased use of rescue medication. Some patients, when they suddenly get worse, will have one puff of the short-acting beta agonist and that is all that is needed to bring them back to normal. The sort of patient I see in hospital practice is sometimes using a whole salbutamol canister every day or two. They're using extra puffs all the time and that clearly reflects the fact that their underlying asthma control is nothing like as good as it ought to be.

Comparison of efficiency of bambuterol and salmeterol

O. Selroos

Mjölbolsta Hospital, Finland, and Department of Clinical R & D,
Astra Draco AB, Lund, Sweden

Summary

The once-daily oral bronchodilator bambuterol and the twice-daily inhaled bronchodilator salmeterol have been compared in only a few studies. In placebo-controlled studies, both bronchodilators have been found clinically effective and with few side-effects. In a double-blind, randomized 6-week parallel-group study in 117 patients with nocturnal asthma and using inhaled or oral steroids, no difference was found in efficacy between bambuterol 20 mg once daily in the evening and salmeterol 50 µg b.i.d. (morning and evening PEF, nocturnal awakenings). Similar results were seen in a double-blind, crossover study in 12 patients comparing 10 mg bambuterol in the evening with salmeterol 50 µg in the evening for 2 weeks each. In a small, double-blind crossover study in 15 patients with reversible airway obstruction, bambuterol 20 mg once daily in the morning was compared with placebo for one week each. The patients were thereafter treated openly for one week with 50 µg salmeterol b.i.d. In steady state, on day 8, the 12- and 24-hour FEV_1 values and the maximum FEV_1 values were not significantly different after treatment with bambuterol or salmeterol. No differences in side-effects were seen. Further comparative double-blind, controlled studies are warranted.

Introduction

Bambuterol hydrochloride (Bambec®, Astra) is the first β_2-agonist with a 24-hour duration of bronchodilatation. It is an oral prodrug of terbutaline, with a considerable presystemic and metabolic stability, designed to be slowly metabolized to terbutaline [1, 2]. It has a similar degree of clinical efficacy to that of other oral bronchodilators, but fewer and milder side-effects, especially with regard to tremor [3–5] (Fig. 1). Placebo-controlled crossover [6] and parallel-group [7] dose-response studies have shown 5 mg once daily to be effective in a few patients, 10 mg once daily to have a clear 24-hour bronchodilatation, and 20 mg once daily to be more effective than 10 mg. In a placebo-controlled study, morning and evening administration of 20 mg bambuterol were compared [8]. Both administrations showed the largest bronchodilatation compared with placebo in the early morning hours. The side-effect profile did not differ between placebo and active treat-

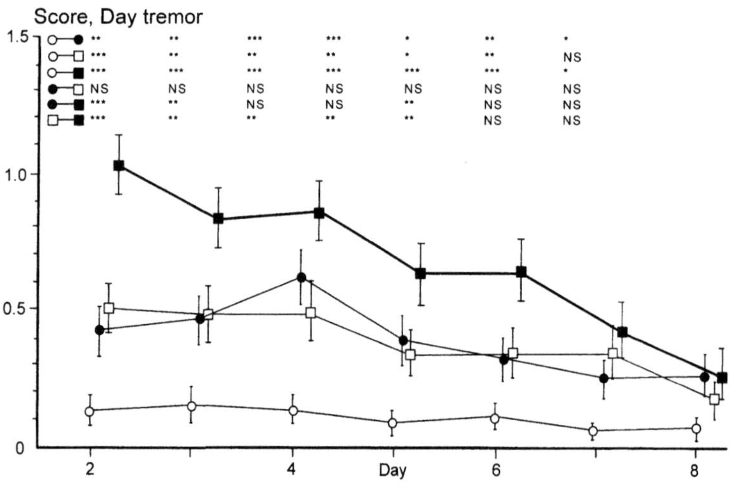

Fig. 1. Daily mean overall tremor score and SEM for the entire treatment week is plotted. * P < 0.05; ** P < 0.01; *** P < 0.001 significance of pairwise comparisons on each day.

○—○ Bambuterol 10 mg; ●—● Bambuterol 20 mg; □—□ Terbutaline CR 5 mg; ■—■ Terbutaline CR 7.5 mg (from ref. [5] with permission)

ments, but evening dosing had fewest side effects. In a placebo-controlled study in 28 patients with nocturnal asthma, evening dosing of 20 mg bambuterol has been found very effective [9].

Salmeterol (Serevent®, Glaxo) is a selective, long-acting inhaled β_2-agonist. It has been found effective in mild to moderate asthma at a dose of 50 μg twice daily [10–13]. In more severe asthma, a dose of 100 μg twice daily was shown to be more effective than 50 μg twice daily in improving lung function and symptom scores [14]. In most instances, however, a dose of 50 μg twice daily has been found sufficient. In a study in patients with nocturnal asthma, salmeterol 50 μg b.i.d. was more effective than the combination of slow-release theophylline and ketotifen [15].

According to current asthma treatment guidelines, long-acting β_2-agonists should not be used for acute symptom relief, but in addition to and on top of anti-inflammatory medication in patients with persisting symptoms [16]. Some patients prefer oral medication; some patients have problems in using inhalers correctly. It is obvious that controlled clinical studies need to be done in order to compare the efficacy and safety of oral bambuterol with those of inhaled salmeterol.

Comparative studies

I. Studies in patients with nocturnal asthma

The effects of a bambuterol tablet, 20 mg in the evening, and of salmeterol pMDI 50 μg b.i.d. were compared in a multicentre study in France comprising a 2-week run-in period and a 6-week double-blind, randomized treatment period [17]. The study had a parallel-group design and a double-dummy blinding technique was used. Terbutaline (Bricanyl® Turbuhaler®) was used as rescue medication. One hundred and seventeen asthmatic patients (65 women, 52 men) aged 20 to 70 years (mean age 45 years) were randomized into the study. They had been on treatment with an inhaled corticosteroid (800–2000 μg per day via a pMDI or 400–2000 μg of budesonide Turbuhaler) or an oral steroid (≤ 20 mg prednisolone per day) for at least 4 weeks before the study. They also had to have a ≥ 15 % overnight fall in their peak expiratory flow (PEF) during at least 3 of the 7 nights of the run-in period, a FEV_1 between 40 and 85 % or predicted normal values and awakening because of asthma symptoms with a need for rescue medication at least once during the run-in period. The patients recorded their PEF values each morning and evening and also the number of nights with awakening due to asthma, and the symptoms and use of rescue medication during day and night. Morning PEF was the primary variable of efficacy. Safety was assessed as subjective tremor scores and reported adverse events.

During the study, the patients continued their treatment with their corticosteroid at an unchanged dose. Fifty-seven patients were randomized to additional treatment with bambuterol. Their baseline mean $FEV_1 \pm SD$ was 1.96 ± 0.58 L corresponding to 64 ± 12 % predicted and the mean reversibility after inhalation of 1.0 mg terbutaline sulphate was 11.2 ± 8.8 %. Sixty patients were randomized to salmeterol. Their baseline mean FEV_1 was 2.00 ± 0.56 L corresponding to 65 ± 13 % predicted and the mean reversibility was 12.5 ± 9.8 %.

The baseline mean morning PEF ± SD was 273 ± 67 L/min in the bambuterol group and 310 ± 80 L/min in the salmeterol group. The changes from baseline were + 28 ± 51 L/min in the bambuterol group and + 29 ± 52 L/min in the salmeterol group. The difference between the groups was not statistically significant.

The evening mean PEF values increased by 20 ± 53 L/min in the bambuterol group and 23 ± 53 L/min in the salmeterol group. The difference between the changes was not statistically significant.

At baseline the percentage of nights per week with nocturnal awakenings was 46 ± 30 in the bambuterol group and 48 ± 30 in the salmeterol group. During the treatment periods, the corresponding figures were 18 ± 25 in the bambuterol group and 25 ± 31 in the salmeterol group. The difference between the changes was not statistically significant.

The mean baseline tremor scores were 0.2 ± 0.5 in the bambuterol group and 0.3 ± 0.6 in the salmeterol group. The corresponding scores during the treatment periods were 0.2 ± 0.3 and 0.2 ± 0.4, respectively. The difference between the changes was not statistically significant.

Five patients reported adverse events during the study which were classified as serious; one in the bambuterol group (asthma deterioration) and four in the salmeterol group (three asthma deteriorations).

This study showed that bambuterol 20 mg in the evening and salmeterol 50 µg b.i.d. were equally effective in patients suffering from night-time asthmatic symptoms despite the use of inhaled corticosteroids.[1]

In a randomized, double-blind, crossover study in 12 patients with nocturnal asthma (age 18–55 years) the patients received bambuterol 10 mg or salmeterol dry powder 50 µg in the evening for 2 weeks each [18]. There was a 7-day wash-out period between the treatments. No significant differences between the treatment were found for mean morning PEF values, nocturnal awakenings or in the use of rescue inhaled terbutaline.

The incidence of drug-related adverse events was low during both treatments and all events were classified as mild. ECG recordings and laboratory tests values were normal.

II. A study in patients with reversible airway obstruction

We performed a two-phase study in 15 asthma patients (7 women, 8 men) with reversible airway obstruction and who had had asthma for a mean of 3.3 ± 2.8 years. Their mean age was 49 years (range 26–67) and their mean reversibility after inhalation of 0.5 mg terbutaline sulphate or 0.2 mg salbutamol was 34 % (range 21–63 %). The first part of the study was a placebo-controlled crossover phase when the patients received either bambuterol 20 mg in the morning or placebo for 1 week each. FEV_1 was measured on the first and the last treatment days hourly for 6 hours and after 9, 12 and 24 hours. In the second part of the study, the patients received 50 µg salmeterol b.i.d. openly for one week, the reason for this design being that we were unable to obtain salmeterol placebo. FEV_1 was measured after the first dose and after the last morning dose at the same time points as after placebo and bambuterol. At 12 and 24 hours, FEV_1 was measured before intake of the next salmeterol dose. PEF was not measured at home.

---

[1] After the presentation of this review another comparative bambuterol-salmeterol study with the same doses has been reported and with similar results (Crompton GK et al. (1997) Thorax 52 [Suppl 6]: A 58).

Baseline mean FEV_1 ± SD on day 1 in the morning before placebo was 2.28 ± 0.72 L, before bambuterol 2.19 ± 0.68 L and before salmeterol 2.31 ± 0.65 L. On day 8, the mean FEV_1 in the morning was 2.32 ± 0.77 L before placebo, 2.30 ± 0.76 L before bambuterol and 2.43 ± 0.64 L before salmeterol treatment.

After the first dose (day 1) there was a mean increase over placebo of 0.13 L 12 hours after intake of bambuterol and of 0.03 L 24 hours after dosing. The mean increase 12 hours after the first dose of 50 μg salmeterol was 0.27 L.

In steady state (day 8) the mean FEV_1 values in the morning and after 12 and 24 hours are shown in Table 1 together with the mean maximum values during the day. At 12 hours, the difference in improvement between bambuterol and placebo was not statistically significant ($p = 0.06$). The same was true of the difference between bambuterol and salmeterol ($p = 0.06$). The difference between placebo and salmeterol was statistically significant ($p = 0.0008$). At 24 hours after dosing (12 hours after inhalation of salmeterol) the difference between bambuterol and placebo was statistically significant ($p = 0.0015$) but not the difference between bambuterol and salmeterol ($p = 0.4728$). The difference between salmeterol and placebo was significant ($p = 0.0003$). When comparing the maximum effects during the 24-hour observation period, no statistically significant difference was seen between the two active treatments ($p = 0.5870$) whereas the differences vs placebo were significant; $p = 0.0009$ for bambuterol vs placebo and $p = 0.0046$ for salmeterol vs placebo.

No serious adverse events occurred during the study. Four instances of mild, transient tremor were reported; one on placebo, one on bambu-

Table 1. Mean ± SD baseline, 12- and 24-hour FEV_1 values and maximum FEV_1 values (L) after one week's treatment (steady state) with placebo, bambuterol 20 mg in the morning and salmeterol 50 μg b.i.d.

	Baseline	12 hours	24 hours	Max value
Placebo	2.32 ± 0.77	2.26 ± 0.74	2.14 ± 0.72	2.50 ± 0.85
Bambuterol	2.30 ± 0.76	2.39 ± 0.76	2.42 ± 0.88	2.72 ± 0.76
Salmeterol	2.43 ± 0.64	2.59 ± 0.73	2.50 ± 0.74	2.78 ± 0.77

terol and two on salmeterol. Palpitations were reported by one patient on placebo treatment.

This study did not show differences in changes in FEV_1 in steady state between bambuterol 20 mg and salmeterol 50 μg b.i.d. in patients with reversible airway obstruction. This result should, however, bc interpreted with caution because only the bambuterol part of the study was blinded, and the number of patients was small.

Conclusion

To the best of our knowledge, results of only three studies comparing the efficacy of oral bambuterol and inhaled salmeterol are available. In these studies in patients with nocturnal asthma and in patients with reversible airway disease, no differences in steady state efficacy or in safety were observed. The preference of using oral or inhaled medication has not been evaluated.

Both bambuterol and salmeterol are long-acting β_2-agonists with maintained bronchodilatation as compared with placebo for 24 and 12 hours respectively. Addition of a long-acting bronchodilator on top of anti-inflammatory medication reduces night-time symptoms and thereby improves the patients' quality of life.

Further double-blind studies comparing the efficacy and safety of oral bambuterol and inhaled salmeterol (and formoterol) are clearly warranted.

References

1. Olsson OAT, Svensson LÅ (1984) New lipophilic terbutaline ester prodrugs with long effect duration. Pharmaceut Res 1: 19–23
2. Svensson LÅ (1987) Bambuterol: a prodrug-prodrug with built-in hydrolysis brake. Acta Pharm Suec 24: 333–341
3. van den Berg W, Alanko K. Sahlström K, Järvinen M, Mikkola E, Jansson C (1989) Bambuterol once every evening 10 mg and 20 mg compared with terbutaline 5 mg three times daily. Eur Respir J 2 [Suppl 8]: 812s
4. Persson G, Pahlm O (1990) Efficacy and safety of bambuterol once daily in comparison with terbutaline t.i.d. Clin Exp Allergy 20 [Suppl 1]: 35
5. Larsen K, Schmekel B (1993) Tremor in healthy volunteers after bambuterol and terbutaline CR-tablets. Eur J Clin Pharmacol 45: 303–305

6. Selroos O, Sahlström K, Backman R, Laxmayr L (1992) Bronchodilating properties of once daily bambuterol in asthma. J Allergy Clin Immunol 89: P339
7. Persson G, Baas A, Knight A, Larsen B, Olsson H (1995) One month treatment with the once daily oral β_2-agonist bambuterol in asthmatic patients. Eur Respir J 8: 34–39
8. D'Alonzo GE, Smolensky MH, Feldman S, Gnosspelius Y, Karlsson K (1995) Bambuterol in the treatment of asthma. A placebo-controlled comparison of once-daily morning vs evening administration. Chest 107: 406–412
9. Petrie GR, Chookang JY, Hassan WU et al (1993) Bambuterol: effective in nocturnal asthma. Respir Med 87: 581–585
10. Ullman A, Svedmyr N (1988) Salmeterol, a new long-acting inhaled β_2-adrenoceptor agonist: a comparison with salbutamol in adult asthmatic patients. Thorax 43: 674–678
11. Dahl R, Earnshaw JS, Palmer JBD (1991) Salmeterol: a four week study of long-acting beta-adrenoceptor agonist for the treatment of reversible airways disease. Eur Respir J 4: 1178–1184
12. Britton MG, Earnshaw JS, Palmer JBD (1992) A twelve month comparison of salmeterol with salbutamol in asthmatic patients. Eur Respir J 5: 1062–1067
13. Pearlman DS, Chervinsky P, LaForce C et al (1992) A comparison of salmeterol with albuterol in the treatment of mild-moderate asthma. N Engl J Med 327: 1420–1425
14. Palmer JBD, Stuart AM, Shepherd GL, Viskum K (1992) Inhaled salmeterol in the treatment of patients with moderate to severe reversible obstructive airways disease – a 3 month comparison of the efficacy and safety of twice daily salmeterol (100 μg) with salmeterol (50 μg). Respir Med 86: 409–417
15. Muir JF, Bertin L, Georges D (1992) Salmeterol versus slow-release theophylline combined with ketotifen in nocturnal asthma: a multicentre trial. Eur Respir J 5: 1197–1200
16. International consensus report on the diagnosis and management of asthma (1992) Clin Exp Allergy 22 [Suppl]: 1–72
17. Wallaert B, Ostinelli J, Arnould B (1995) Long acting β_2 agonists: a comparison of oral bambuterol and inhaled salmeterol in asthmatic patients with nocturnal symptoms. Eur Respir J 8 [Suppl 19]: 1s
18. Justicia JL, Segurado E, Munos MA et al (1995) Salmeterol versus bambuterol in nocturnal asthma. Allergy 50 [Suppl 26]: 315

Correspondence: Prof. Dr. Olof Selroos, Box 34, S-22100 Lund, Sweden.

Discussion

Dr. Fabbri: Thank you for this very clear presentation. The data are certainly very convincing. I mean, they are very interesting and I think they have not been properly evaluated within the guidelines. And the only rationale for recommending the inhaled route was that the data available showed that oral administration or systemic administration in any case, was associated with more side effects. You just showed some data on the side effects and convinced me that they are no different. What about the others?

Dr. Selroos: We discussed this yesterday, when Professor Svensson showed the preclinical profile and the rationale for the prodrug principle, why we don't see side effects after oral dosing of bambuterol. I think I can refer to that discussion.

Dr. Kummer: So the compliance was, in fact, better with the tablet or was this just an assumption?

Dr. Selroos: We have not looked upon that specifically in the study. It was my personal suggestion that, maybe, compliance can be better but we don't know.

Dr. Fabbri: There is a paper suggesting a better compliance with oral drugs. Kelloway et al. (Archives of Internal Medicine, 1994, 154:1349) were taking data from files of the Health Maintenance Organisation, and they could show that the compliance with theophylline was in the range of 50 to 70 per cent, depending on the two age groups. The compliance with inhaled steroids was in the 30 to 50% range, and the compliance with cromoline was in the 20–40% range. So there is at least one reference. Even if these data are taken from records, they do suggest that indeed oral medication is associated with better compliance.

Dr. Selroos: There is also a bambuterol study in the elderly, showing that the use of tablets is easier than that of inhalers.

Dr. Anderson: Does bambuterol or any of its daughter products cross the blood-brain barrier? Is there any effect on quality of sleep?

Dr. Greening: There must be a higher sustained plasma level of this drug in comparison to the inhaled drugs. That's an interesting point of discussion.

Dr. Selroos: The plasma concentration of formed terbutaline is low compared to the concentration after administration of plain terbutaline tablets, but higher than after inhalation.

Dr. Anderson: And of the many daughter products as well?

Dr. Svensson: They don't cross the blood-brain barrier, neither bambuterol nor the metabolites. As bambuterol is an amphiphilic compound, it's not fat-soluble enough to cross the blood-brain barrier.

The future of relievers and controllers in asthma therapy

A. Papi, B. Beghé, G. Caramori,
A. Ciaccia and *L. M. Fabbri*

Institute of Respiratory Diseases, University of Ferrara, Italy*

Summary

Treatment of persistent asthma with anti-inflammatory and bronchodilator agents will probably remain in the first line treatment for at least the next 5 years. The only 2 new options that might become available in the next five years are: a) the use of long-acting bronchodilators, and particularly inhaled salmeterol and formoterol, alone or in combination with very low dose inhaled glucocorticoids; and/or b) cysteinyl-leukotrienes receptor-antagonists and synthesis-inhibitors. Also the pharmacologic treatment of asthma exacerbations will not probably change significantly in the near future.

Introduction

For many years asthma has been defined by its symptoms, reversible airflow limitation, and airway hyperresponsivenes [1]. According to this definition, the cornerstone agents for the treatment of asthma have been

* Supported by: MURST (fondi 60% e 40%), Ferrararicerche, and European Community (Project -Enfumosa- as part of the Project Biomed 2).

bronchodilators. The "Global Initiative for Asthma", a document prepared by a panel of experts convened by the National Institute of Health and the World Health Organization has recently proposed a substantially different definition of asthma, mainly based on pathology and its functional consequences. This definition recognizes that asthma is associated with a chronic inflammation of the airways and that variations of the clinical activity of the disease are associated with variations of the degree and type of airway inflammation [2].

Based on the functional consequences of airway inflammation, the following definition of asthma has been proposed: Asthma is a chronic inflammatory disorder of the airways, in which many cells play a role, in particular eosinophils, mast cells, and T lymphocytes. In susceptible individuals this inflammation causes recurrent episodes of wheezing, breathlessness, chest tightness, and cough, particularly at night and in the early morning. These symptoms are usually associated with widespread but variable airflow limitation that is at least partly reversible, either spontaneously or with treatment. The airway inflammation also causes an associated increase in airway responsiveness to a variety of stimuli. This definition recognizes that asthma is associated with a chronic inflammation of the airways and that variations of the clinical activity of the disease are associated with variations of the degree and type of airway inflammation. According to these concepts, airway inflammation is considered to be the cause of airway hyperresponsiveness, and symptoms and airflow limitation are considered the clinical consequences of the underlying airway inflammation and hyperresponsiveness [2]. These guidelines suggest that the main aim of asthma management is to put and to maintain asthma under control, i.e. to reduce symptoms and asthma exacerbations.

Present approach to the pharmacological treatment of asthma

Pharmacological control of asthma may be obtained in most asthmatics with anti-inflammatory agents (*controllers*), particularly inhaled glucocorticoids [2]. In addition to anti-inflammatory agents, although to a lesser degree, long-acting β_2-agonists (e.g. inhaled salmeterol or formoterol; oral bambuterol, slow release terbutaline) and sustained-release theophylline have also been shown to put and maintain asthma under control, but, at variance with inhaled glucocorticoids [3–7], do not reverse airway inflammation and hyperresponsiveness. Controllers do not rapidly reverse the acute manifestations of asthma [2].

By contrast, short-acting bronchodilators rapidly reverse the acute manifestations of asthma, i.e. respiratory symptoms and airflow limitation, and for this reason they are named *relievers* [2].

The current guidelines recommend that whenever asthma is persistent, in addition to a major effort to prevent asthma by instructing the patients to avoid triggers, pharmacological treatment should include 1) regular anti-inflammatory agents (inhaled glucocorticoids, cromones, slow release theophylline and oral glucocorticoids only in severe patients) plus, 2) short acting bronchodilators only where needed [2]. In addition, the guidelines recommend 3) regular treatment with long-acting bronchodilators, and particularly inhaled salmeterol or formoterol, when regular anti-inflammatory agents do not put and/or maintain asthma under control.

Long-acting bronchodilators, and particularly inhaled salmeterol or formoterol, have been shown to put and maintain asthma under clinical control also without the need of an anti-inflammatory agent but, at variance with inhaled glucocorticoids, they do not prevent asthma exacerbations and do not reverse airway inflammation and hyperresponsiveness [8–10]. Recent studies have reported some anti-inflammatory effect of low dose theophylline [7, 11–13] and for these reasons, at the present time, long-acting inhaled β_2-agonists alone are not recommended in the maintenance treatment of asthma [2, 10], however their use is recommended early in addition to an ineffective dose of inhaled glucocorticoids steroid because the association between a long-acting inhaled β_2-agonist with inhaled glucocorticoids is more effective than increasing the dose of inhaled glucocorticoids. In fact, three recent studies have clearly shown that the addition of salmeterol to an ineffective dose of inhaled glucocorticoid is more efficacious in controlling asthma as compared with the doubling of the dose of inhaled glucocorticoid [14–16]. Based on this evidence, the place of long-acting inhaled β_2-agonists in the maintenance treatment of asthma is in association with inhaled glucocorticoids in mild-moderate persistent asthma not controlled by the recommended dose of inhaled glucocorticoids [2]. Further, because long-acting inhaled β_2-agonists have a long lasting protective effect against exercise-induced asthma in adults, one additional recommendation for their use is the occasional prolonged protection from exercise-induced asthma [17].

The treatment of asthma exacerbations is purely symptomatic, and is based prevalently on the administration of oxygen, short-acting bronchodilators and systemic glucocorticoids [2]. Short-acting inhaled β_2-agonists are usually the preferred bronchodilators used in the treatment of asthma exacerbations [2] but, if there is no prompt response, the addition of an anticholinergic can be useful [18]. Repetitive administration of inhaled short-acting $\beta_2$agonists, rapidly reverses acute airflow limitation [2]. Nebulized salbutamol is the most effective and safest treatment for patients with asthma exacerbations treated either on route to hospital by emergency ambulance personnel or in the emergency room [19, 20]. High dose salbutamol administered from a metered-dose inhaler connected to a spacer may be as effective as nebulized high dose salbutamol [21]. In hypercapnic severe asthma exacerbations, nebulized salbutamol has a greater efficacy and fewer side effects than intravenous salbutamol [22].

Despite the consolidated clinical practice, the role of aminophylline in the treatment of asthma exacerbations appear to be secondary. Intravenous aminophylline is not recommended in the emergency department within the first 4 hours of treatment: however, it may have a role in the treatment of patients hospitalized with severe asthma exacerbations [23–28].

Magnesium sulfate does not seem useful in the treatment of asthma exacerbations [29].

New agents that might change the approach to the pharmacological treatment of asthma in the next 5 years

Relievers

It is likely that the actual approach to the pharmacological treatment of asthma exacerbations, i.e inhaled β_2-agonist in association with oral glucocorticoids, which is very simple and effective, will last long. However, preliminary data are available showing new indications for some antiasthma drugs.

For example, some studies suggest that, in mild asthma exacerbations, the more potent inhaled glucocorticoids (fluticasone and budesonide) are as effective as systemic glucocorticoids [30–33].

At the present time, long-acting inhaled β_2-agonists are not recommended for the treatment of asthma exacerbations, but because of formoterol's rapid onset of action equal to salbutamol [34] it might be interesting to study its potential role in the treatment of asthma exacerbations.

Although inhaled anticholinergics alone have no role in the treatment of asthma exacerbations, in some patients the combination of nebulized ipratropium bromide with salbutamol or fenoterol may produce greater bronchodilation than either drug alone [35–41] or, even if it does not improve the maximal bronchodilator response to salbutamol, it may increase the duration of its bronchodilator response [38]. Oxitropium bromide is a new inhaled anticholinergic with efficacy equal or superior to ipratropium bromide but it has a more rapid onset and prolonged action [42]. It will be interesting to study the combination between nebulized oxitropium bromide and inhaled short-acting β_2-agonists in the treatment of asthma exacerbations.

Controllers

The present pharmacological treatment of persistent asthma is mainly limited by the lack of long-term prospective studies, providing evidence of its efficacy on the natural history of the disease in the absence of any side-effects [2]. There is some concern on the potential side-effects associated with the prolonged use of both regular short-acting β_2-agonists [43] in patients with persistent asthma, and/either systemic or high dose inhaled glucocorticoids particularly in subjects at risk (children, postmenopausal women) [8, 44].

Present regimes recommend the use of inhaled drugs, which maximize clinical effectiveness and minimize side-effects [2]. However, the main limitations of inhaled drugs are the incorrect inhalation methods [45] and the poor compliance of the patients [46].

Methotrexate, cyclosporin A and other systemic glucocorticoids sparing drugs remain experimental agents, and should be used only in selected patients under the supervision of an asthma specialist with previous experimental experience [47].

The cysteinyl-leukotrienes mediate a number of pathways relevant to the pathogenesis of asthma including increased mucus secretion, increased vascular permeability, and smooth muscle contraction and can play a role in maintaining the chronic inflammatory response [48–50]. Cysteinyl-leukotrienes receptor antagonists and leukotriene synthesis-inhibitors are probably the only class of antiasthma agents that might become available in the next 5 years. Indeed, these drugs are clinically effective in asthma [51–54] and seem to have anti-inflammatory action [55, 56], but further comparative studies, in particular with inhaled glucocorticoids, are necessary to understand their exact role. More interestingly these agents might also represent an important adjunct therapy in patients who fail to respond to high dose inhaled glucocorticoids or systemic glucocorticoids [57].

At variance with cysteinyl-leukotrienes receptors antagonists, leukotriene B_4-receptor antagonists do not appear promising antiasthma agents [58].

Although the exact molecular mechanism of action of theophylline is not fully understood, it is known that theophylline is a non-selective inhibitor of intracellular phosphodiesterase (PDE) [59]. Different iso-enzymes of phosphodiesterase are selectively expressed in specific cell types, and recently selective PDE-iso-enzyme inhibitors have been developed [59]. PDE III (smooth muscle) and PDE IV (inflammatory cells, smooth muscle cells) inhibitors are currently under investigation for the treatment of asthma [59]. As compared to theophylline, PDE IV and possibly mixed PDE III and IV inhibitors may have a more selective and specific anti-inflammatory action in asthma [59]. The clinical efficacy of these compounds have not been yet clearly shown.

Other new potentially controllers for asthma treatment include combination of inhaled loop-diuretics with acetylsalicilic acid [60] and selective tachykinins or kinins receptor antagonists [61–63].

In patients with allergic asthma, the treatment with humanised monoclonal antibodies directed against the cristalizable fragment (Fc) of immunoglobulin E (IgE) reduces serum levels of IgE, but not symptoms [64, 65].

Because nitric oxide might act as an inflammatory mediator in asthma [66-68], specific inducible nitric oxide synthase (iNOS) inhibitors [68], may represent potential anti-inflammatory agents [69].

Platelet-activating factor (PAF) has been proposed as an important inflammatory mediator in asthma, but PAF antagonists have never been shown to have a clinically relevant effect in asthma [70, 71], and thus do not appear promising controllers.

The available antihistamines, serotonin receptor antagonists and potassium channel openers do not appear promising controllers, however some preliminary data have shown promising results of the combination of antihistamines and cysteinyl-leukotrienes receptors antagonists [72–76].

Many cytokines are implicated in the pathogenesis of asthma [77–83], and many studies are yet necessary to clarify the hypothetical role in asthma of cytokines as drug target (cytokine-receptor antagonists, cytokine-receptor agonists, cytokine synthesis/secretion inhibitors and circulating cytokine-receptors analogues) [84].

Recent advances in the genetics of atopy, bronchial hyperresponsiveness and asthma [85] could provide gene therapy of asthma as a future treatment.

References

1. American Thoracic Society Committee on Diagnostic Standards for Non tuberculous Respiratory Diseases (1962). Definition and classification of chronic bronchitis, asthma, and pulmonary emphysema. Am Rev Respir Dis 85: 762–768
2. Sheffer AL (ed) Global Initiative for Asthma. NHLBI/WHO Workshop report. National Institutes of Health, National Heart, Lung and Blood Institute. Publication No. 95-3659. January 1995
3. Booth H, Richmond I, Ward C, Gardiner PV, Harkawat R, Walters EH (1995) Effect of high dose inhaled fluticasone propionate on airway inflammation in asthma. Am J Respir Crit Care Med 152: 45–52

4. Haahtela T, Jarvinen M, Kava T, Kiviranta K, Koskinen S, Lehtonen K, Nikander K, Persson T, Reinikainen K, Selroos O, Sovijarvi A, Stenius-Aarniala B, Svahn T, Tammivaara R, Laitinen LA (1991) Comparison of a beta$_2$-agonist, terbutaline, with an inhaled corticosteroid, budesonide, in newly detected asthma. N Engl J Med 325: 388–392
5. Trigg CJ, Manolitsas ND, Wang J, Calderòn MA, McAulay A, Jordan SE, Herdman MJ, Jhalli N, Duddle JM, Hamilton SA, Devalia JL, Davies RJ (1994) Placebo-controlled immunopathologic study of four months of inhaled corticosteroids in asthma. Am J Respir Crit Care Med 150: 17–22.
6. Manolitsas ND, Wang J, Devalia JL, Trigg CJ, McAulay AE, Davies RJ (1995) Regular albuterol, nedocromil sodium, and bronchial inflammation in asthma. Am J Respir Crit Care Med 151: 1925–1930
7. Djukanovic R, Finnerty JP, Lee C, Wilson S, Madden J, Holgate ST (1995) The effects of theophylline on mucosal inflammation in asthmatic airways: biopsy results. Eur Respir J 8: 831–833
8. Barnes PJ (1995) Inhaled glucocorticoids for asthma. N Engl J Med 332: 868–875
9. Gardiner PV, Ward C, Booth H, Allison A, Hendrick DJ, Walters EH (1994) Effects of eight weeks of treatment with salmeterol on bronchoalveolar lavage inflammatory indices in asthmatics. Am J Respir Crit Care Med 150: 1006–1011
10. Nelson HS (1995) Drug therapy: β-adrenergic bronchodilators. N Engl J Med 333: 499–506
11. Finnerty JP, Lee C, Wilson S, Madden J, Djukanovic R, Holgate ST (1996) Effects of theophylline on inflammatory cells and cytokines in asthmatic subjects: a placebo-controlled parallel group study. Eur Respir J 9: 1672–1677
12. Sullivan P, Bekir S, Jaffar Z, Page CP, Jeffery P, Costello J (1994) Anti-inflammatory effects of low-dose oral theophylline in atopic asthma. Lancet 343: 1006–1008
13. Weinberger M, Hendeles L (1996) Theophylline in asthma. N Engl J Med 334: 1380–1388
14. Greening AP, Ind PW, Northfield M, Shaw G, on behalf of Allen and Hanburys Limited UK Study Group (1994) Added salmeterol versus higher-dose corticosteroid in asthma patients with symptoms on existing inhaled corticosteroid. Lancet 344: 219–224
15. Woolcock A, Lundback B, Ringdal OLN, Jacques LA (1996) Comparison of addition of salmeterol to inhaled steroids with doubling of the dose of inhaled steroids. Am J Respir Crit Care Med 153: 1481–1488
16. Faurschou P, Steffensen I, Jacques L, European Respiratory Group (1996) Effect of addition of inhaled salmeterol to the moderate-to-severe asthmatics uncontrolled on high-dose inhaled steroids. Eur Respir J 9: 1885–1890
17. Kemp JP, Dockhorn J, Busse WW, Bleecker ER, van As A (1994)

Prolonged effect of inhaled salmeterol against exercise-induced bronchospasm. Am J Respir Crit Care Med 150: 1612–1615
18. Karpell JP, Schacter EN, Fanta C, Levey D, Spiro P, Aldric T, Menjoge SS, Witex TJ (1996) A comparison of ipratropium and albuterol vs albuterol alone for the treatment of acute asthma. Chest 110: 611–616
19. Campbell IA, Colman SB, Mao JH, Prescott RJ, Weston CFM (1995) An open, prospective comparison of beta$_2$-agonists given via nebuliser, Nebuhaler, or pressurised inhaler by ambulance crew as emergency treatment. Thorax 50: 79–80
20. Fergusson RJ, Stewart CM, Wathen CG, Moffat R, Crompton GK (1995) Effectiveness of nebulised salbutamol administered in ambulances to patients with severe acute asthma. Thorax 50: 81–82
21. Idris AH, McDermott MF, Raucci JC, Morrabel A, McGorray S, Hendeles L (1993) Emergency Department treatment of severe asthma: metered-dose inhaler plus holding chamber is equivalent in effectiveness to nebulizer. Chest 103: 665–672
22. Salmeron S, Brochard L, Mal H, Tenaillon A, Henry-Amar M, Renon D, Duroux P, Simonneau G (1994) Nebulized versus intravenous albuterol in hypercapnic acute asthma: a multicenter, double–blind, randomized study. Am J Respir Crit Care Med 149: 1466–1470
23. Coleridge J, Cameron P, Epstein J, Teichtahl H (1993) Intravenous aminophylline confers no benefit in acute asthma treated with intravenous steroids and inhaled bronchodilators. Aust N Z J Med 23: 348–354
24. Huang D, O'Brien RG, Harman E, Aull L (1993) Does aminophylline benefit adults admitted to the hospital for an acute exacerbation of asthma. Ann Intern Med 119: 1155–1160
25. Janson C, Boman G, Boe J (1992) Which patients benefit from adding theophylline to beta$_2$-agonist treatment in severe acute asthma?. Ann Allergy 69: 107–110
26. Murphy DG, McDermott MF, Rydman RJ, Sloan EP, Zalenski RJ (1993) Aminophylline in the treatment of acute asthma when beta$_2$-adrenergics agents and steroids are provided. Arch Intern Med 153: 1784–1788
27. Rodrigo C, Rodrigo R (1994) Treatment of acute asthma: lack of therapeutic benefit and increase of the toxicity from aminophylline given in addition to high doses of salbutamol delivered by metered-dose inhaler with a spacer. Chest 106: 1071–1076
28. Zainudin BMZ, Ismail O, Yusoff K (1994) Effect of adding aminophylline infusion to nebulised salbutamol in severe acute asthma. Thorax 49: 267–269
29. Skorodin MS (1995) Magnesium in pulmonary and critical care medicine. Clin Pulm Med 2: 231–237
30. Levy ML, Stevenson C, Maslen T (1996) Comparison of short courses of oral prednisolone and fluticasone propionate in the treatment of adults

with acute exacerbations of asthma in primary care. Thorax 51: 1087–1092
31. Lim TK (1996) Comparison of inhaled fluticasone propionate and oral prednisolone in the treatment of acute severe asthma. Am J Respir Care Med 153 [Suppl]: A340
32. Morice AH, Morris D, Lawson-Mattehew (1995) Nebulised budesonide in acute severe asthma. Am J Respir Care Med 151 [Suppl]: A274
33. Praparn Y, Maranetra N, Nana A, Charoenratanakul S, Boe J, Lofdahl C-G, Selroos O, Stahl E (1995) Inhaled as effective as oral steroids after an acute asthma attack. Am J Respir Care Med 151 [Suppl]: A274
34. van Noord JA, Smeets JJ, Raaijmakers JAM, Bommer AM, Maesen FPV (1996) Salmeterol versus formoterol in patients with moderately severe asthma: onset and duration of action. Eur Respir J 9: 1684–1688
35. Rebuck AS, Chapman KR, Abboud R, Pare PD, Kreisman H, Wolkove N, Vickerson F (1987) Nebulized anticholinergic and sympathomimetic treatment of asthma and chronic obstructive airways disease in the emergency room. Am J Med 82: 59–64
36. O'Driscoll BR, Taylor RJ, Horsley MG, Chambers DK, Bernstein A (1989) Nebulised salbutamol with and without ipratropium bromide in acute airflow obstruction. Lancet 2: 1418–1420
37. Bryant DH (1985) Nebulized ipratropium bromide in the treatment of acute asthma. Chest 88: 24–29
38. Higgins RM, Stradling JR, Lane DJ (1988) Should ipratropium bromide be added to beta-agonists in treatment of acute severe asthma? Chest 94: 718–722
39. Leahy BC, Gomm SA, Allen SC (1983) Comparison of nebulised salbutamol with nebulised ipratropium bromide in acute asthma. Br J Dis Chest 77: 159–163
40. Summers QA, Tarala RA (1990) Nebulised ipratropium in the treatment of acute asthma. Chest 97: 430–434
41. Ward MJ, McFarlane JT, Davies D (1985) A place for ipratropium bromide in the treatment of severe acute asthma. Br J Dis Chest 79: 374–378
42. Bauer R (1992) The pharmacology of oxitropium bromide. Rev Contemp Pharmocoter 3: 197–203
43. Crane J, Pearce N, Burgess C, Beasley R (1995) Asthma and the β-agonist debate. Thorax 50 [Suppl 1]: S5–S10
44. Barnes PJ, Pedersen S (1993) Efficacy and safety of inhaled corticosteroids in asthma. Am Rev Respir Dis 148 [Suppl]: S1–S26
45. Matthys H (1990) Inhalation delivery of asthma drugs. Lung [Suppl]: 645–652
46. Kelloway JS, Wyatt RA, Adlis SA (1994) Comparison of patients'compliance with prescribed oral and inhaled asthma medications. Arch Intern Med 154: 1349–1352
47. Fabbri L, Caramori G, Cosma P, Ciaccia A (1996) Methotrexate in the treat-

ment of systemic glucocorticoid dependent severe persistent astma: a word of caution. Monaldi Archiv Chest Dis 51: 130–137

48. Dahlèn B, Dahlèn S-E (1995) Leukotrienes as mediators of airway obstruction and inflammation in asthma. Clin Exp Allergy 25 [Suppl 2]: 50–54
49. Laitinen LA, Laitinen A, Haahtela T, Vilkka V, Spur BW, Lee TH (1993) Leukotriene E_4 and granulocytic infiltration into asthmatic airways. Lancet 341: 989–990
50. Stechschulte DJ (1990) Leukotrienes in asthma and allergic rhinitis. N Engl J Med 323: 1769–1770
51. Israel E, Rubin P, Kemp JP, Grossman J, Pierson W, Siegal SC, Tinkelman D, Murray JJ, Busse W, Segal AT, Fish J, Kaiser HB, Ledford D, Wenzel S, Rosenthal R, Cohn J, Lanni C, Pearlman H, Karahalios P, Drazen JM (1993) The effect of inhibition of 5-lipoxygenase by zileuton in mild to moderate asthma. Ann Intern Med 119: 1059–1066
52. Israel E, Cohn J, Dibè L, Drazen MJ, for the Zileuton Clinical Trial Group (1996) Effect of treatment with zileuton, a 5-lipoxygenase inhibitor, in patients with asthma: a randomized clinical trial. J Am Med Assoc 275: 931–936
53. Meltzer SS, Hasday JD, Cohn J, Bleecker ER (1996) Inhibition of exercise-induced bronchospasm by zileuton: a 5-lipoxygenase inhibitor. Am J Respir Crit Care Med 153: 931–935
54. Spector SL, Smith LJ, Glass M and the Accolate™ Asthma trialists Group (1994) Effects of 6 weeks of therapy with oral doses of ICI 204,219, a leukotriene D_4 receptor antagonist in subjects with bronchial asthma. Am J Respir Crit Care Med 150: 618–623
55. Kane GC, Pollice M, Kim CJ, Cohn J, Dworski RT, Murray JJ, Sheller JR, Fish JE, Peters SP (1996) A controlled trial of the effect of the 5-lipoxygenase inhibitor, zileuton, on lung inflammation produced by segmental antigen challenge in human beings. J Allergy Clin Immunol 97: 646–654
56. Wenzel SE, Trudeau JB, Kaminsky DA, Cohn J, Martin RJ, Westcott JY (1995) Effect of 5-lipoxygenase inhibition on bronchoconstriction and airway inflammation in nocturnal asthma. Am J Respir Crit Care Med 152: 897–905
57. Ikeda K, Obata H, Fujita H, Nahanishi T, Tsuruta R (1996) Pranlukast (ONO-1078, leukotriene receptor antagonist) enabled to reduce steroid doses in chronic severe adult asthma. Chest 110 [Suppl]: 88s abstract
58. Evans DJ, Barnes PJ, Spaethe MS, van Alstyne EL, Mitchell M, O'Connor BJ (1996) Effect of a leukotriene B_4 Receptor antagonist, LY293111, on allergen induced responses in asthma. Thorax 51: 1178–1184
59. Banner KH, Page CP (1995) Theophylline and selective phosphodiesterase inhibitors as anti-inflammatory drugs in the treatment of bronchial asthma. Eur Respir J 8: 996–1000
60. Bianco S, Vaghi A, Robuschi M, Refini RM, Pieroni MG, Sestini P (1995)

Steroid-sparing effect of inhaled lysine acetylsalicylate and furosemide in high-dose beclomethasone-dependent asthma. J Allergy Clin Immunol 95: 937–943
61. Ichinose M, Miura M, Yamauchi H, Kageyama N, Tomaki M, Oyake T, Ohuchi Y, Hida W, Miki H, Tamura G, Shirato K (1996) A neurokinin 1-receptor antagonist improves exercise-induced airway narrowing in asthmatic patients. Am J Respir Crit Care Med 153: 936–941
62. Regoli D, Boudon A, Fauchère J-L (1994) Receptors and antagonists for substance P and related peptides. Pharmacol Rev 46: 551–599
63. Bertrand C, Geppetti P (1996) Tachykinin and kinin receptor antagonist: therapeutic prospectives in allergic airway disease. Trends Pharmacol Sci 17: 255–259
64. Fahy JV, Fleming HE, Wong HH, Liu JT, Su JQ, Reimann J, Fick RB, Boushey HA (1996) The effect of treatment with a monoclonal antibody directed against IgE on allergic airway response in asthmatic subjects. J Allergy Clin Immunol 97: 358, abstract 702
65. Cockcroft DW, Kalra S, Bhagat R, Swystum VA, Boulet L-P, Cote J, Laviolette M, Deschesnes F, Chapman KR, Cleland LD, Fick RB, Su J, De Vault A (1996) rhuMAb-E25(E25), humanized murine monoclonal anti-IgE, inhibits the allergen-induced early asthmatic response (EAR). J Allergy Clin Immunol 97: 315, abstract 532
66. Massaro AF, Gaston B, Kita D, Fanta C, Stamler JS, Drazen JM (1995) Expired nitric oxide levels during treatment of acute asthma. Am J Respir Crit Care Med 152: 800–803
67. Lunderberg JON, Weitzberg E, Lunderberg JM, Alving K (1996) Nitric oxide in exhaled air. Eur Respir J 9: 2671–2680
68. Yates DH, Kharitonov SA, Thomas PS, Barnes PJ (1996) Endogenous nitric oxide is decreased in asthmatic patients by an inhibitor of inducible nitric oxide synthase. Am J Respir Crit Care Med 154: 247–250
69. Barnes PJ, Liew FY (1995) Nitric oxide and asthmatic inflammation. Immunol Today 16: 128–130
70. Kuitert LM, Angus RM, Barnes NC, Barnes PJ, Bone MF, Chung KF, Fairfax AJ, Higenbotham TW, O'Connor BJ, Piotrowska B, Rozniecki J, Uden S, Walters EH, Willard CJ (1995) Effect of a novel potent platelet-activating factor antagonist, modipafant, in clinical asthma. Am J Respir Crit Care Med 151: 1331–1335
71. Spencer DPS, Johnston SL, Calverley PMA, Dhillon P, Higging C, Ramhamadany E, Turner S, Winning A, Winter J, Holgate ST (1994) The effect of the orally active platelet-activating factor antagonist WEB 2086 in the treatment of asthma. Am J Respir Crit Care Med 149: 1142–1148
72. Cazzola M, Matera MG, D'Amato G, Rossi F (1995) Effects of serotonin on airways: recent developments. Allergy 50: 1–10
73. Faurschou P, Mikkelsen KL, Steffensen I, Franke B (1994) The lack of

bronchodilator effect and the short-term safety of cumulative single doses of an inhaled potassium channel opener (bimakalim) in adult patients with mild to moderate bronchial asthma. Pulm Pharmacol 7: 293–297
74. Spector S, Miller CJ, Glass M (1995) 13-week dose-response study with accolate™ (zafirlukast) in patients with mild to moderate asthma. Am J Respir Crit Care Med 151 [Suppl]: A379
75. Williams AJ, Lee TH, Cochrane GM, Hopkirk A, vyse T, Chiew F, Lavender E, Richards DH, Owen S, Stone P, Church S, Woodcock AA (1990) Attenuation of nocturnal asthma by cromakalim. Lancet 336: 334–336
76. Dahlen S-E (1996) Personal comunication to L. Fabbri
77. Casale TB, Costa JJ, Galli SJ (1996) TNFα is important in human lung allergic reactions. Am J Respir Cell Mol Biol 15: 35-44
78. Cruikshank WW, Long A, Tarpy RE, Kornfeld H, Caroll M, Teran L, Holgate ST, Center DM (1995) Early identification of interleukin-16 (lymphocyte chemoattractant factor) and macrophage inflammatory protein 1α (MIP1α) in bronchoalveolar lavage fluid of antigen-challenged asthmatics. Am J Respir Cell Mol Biol 13: 738–747
79. Egan RW, Umland SP, Cuss FM, Chapman RW (1996) Biology of interleukin-5 and its relevance to allergic disease. Allergy 51: 71–81
80. Kips JC, Brusselle GJ, Joos GF, Peleman RA, Tavernier JA, Devos RR, Pauwels RA (1996) Interleukin-12 inhibits antigen-induced airway hyperresponsiveness in mice. Am J Respir Crit Care Med 153: 535–539
81. Moller MG, de Jong TAW, van der Kwast TH, Overbeek SE, Wierenga-Wolf AF, Thepen T, Hoogsteden HC (1996) Immunolocalization of interleukin-4 in eosinophils in the bronchial mucosa of atopic asthmatics. Am J Respir Cell Mol Biol 14: 439–443
82. Robinson DS, Tsicopoulos A, Meng Q, Durham SM, Kay BA, Hamid Q (1996) Increased interleukin-10 messenger RNA expression in atopic allergy and asthma. Am J Respir Cell Mol Biol 14: 113–117
83. Teran LM, Davies DE (1996) The chemokines: their potential role in allergic inflammation. Clin Exp Allergy 26: 1005–1019
84. van Oosterhout AJM, Savelkoul HFJ (1995) Interleukin 5 as a drug target in allergy and asthma. Trends Pharmacol Sci 16: 37
85. Sandford A, Weir T, Parè P (1996) The genetics of asthma. Am J Respir Crit Care Med 153: 1749–1765

Correspondence: Alberto Papi, Laboratorio di Ricerca su Asma e BPCO, Università di Ferrara, Via Savonarola, 9, I-44100 Ferrara, Italy.

Discussion

Dr. Fabbri: I wanted just to give the general perspectives. So please feel free to discuss any of the presentations of this session now.

Dr. Selroos: I have a comment with reference to the study we published with Haahthela as the first author. You mentioned that in that study we also showed that when stopping treatment asthma comes back. But that's not the full truth. After two years' treatment with budesonide, the patients were randomised to a lower dose of budesonide or to placebo. What happened in the placebo group was that we had three almost equally big sub-groups. One third of the patients deteriorated immediately, one third by the end of this follow-up year, but one third of the patients did not develop asthma symptoms or abnormal airway function and they remained with regard to hyper-responsiveness within the normal level during one year on placebo. So there was a small sub-group of patients who did not deteriorate when they had had early treatment, and when they had had symptoms for less than twelve months after starting treatment.

Dr. Fabbri: Thank you for your comment. I was just pooling together the data, particularly yours and those of Juniper. However, if you look carefully at the genetic study published by D. Postma et al. (NEJM 1995, 333: 894–900) for the chromosome 5 association, you see that in the long-term follow-up of patients, you have some asthmatics without considering treatment because they just have remission. So I'm sure you would be reluctant to think that those 10 or 15 asymptomatic patients would be so even without treatment. It's a chance, you might have full remission. The suggestion is that probably by taking steroids very early, you increase the chances to have this full remission of some of the patients.

Dr. Boyd: I think you're making a very important point. Because whenever we change the balance of treatment, where we're adding things to people on inhaled steroid therapy, we are assuming that they are all responding. And it's really quite a long time ago, we published a paper looking at twice daily as opposed to four times daily regimes with BDP and we selected out the patients who responded or who did not respond by stopping the inhaled steroid and identifying those who did not deteriorate as opposed to those who did. I think it's a problem with all clinical trial work, that we have to be confident, that we know that the patients required treatment or are responding to the therapy we give them in the way we expect. And I think there is a proportion of people on inhaled steroid therapy who apparently clinically don't require it.

Dr. Rudolf: We're clearly getting to the time of day where we're making philosophical points. But I wonder if I could ask your view about what I think is an important issue, that is precisely what we actually call the drugs in general terms, especially when we're trying to educate non-specialists and patients on how to use their drugs. At one time, it was easy. We had relievers, the short-acting beta-agonists, and what were called preventers, which were by and large the inhaled steroids and the cromones. I recollect that when the long-acting inhaled beta-agonists first appeared, they were referred to as controllers. But now we're seeing the term controllers being used to include what certainly I and many other people still regard as the true preventers. So I'd like your view on that.

The second point, and this came out briefly in discussion yesterday, was the use of the words inflammation and anti-inflammatory. I think that the degree of inflammation varies a lot from patient to patient. So far as the so-called anti-inflammatory drugs are concerned, we know that some drugs work in some patients but not others. I think that calling them all anti-inflammatory drugs is not necessarily right, and I'm unhappy with calling them all controllers. We know that for theophyllines the suggested word has been immunomodulatory. But all these new drugs, the leukotriene antagonists and the anti-interleukins and so on, what should we call these drugs?

Dr. Fabbri: Well, we'd better learn first what they do and then decide. But I tell you, my broken English would not allow me to speculate on the best word. So you can do it within the UK community.

But I would like to go back to one of the points that came up in the discussion before. Dr. Boyd, you raised the point, your patient leaves the medication. Let me try to put it provocatively. Now suppose that we accept, that long-acting beta-agonists must be taken together with the steroids. Nevertheless, we are speculating, wether this clinical practice has to be maintained. You have convincingly shown in two studies that the number of exacerbations did not increase and the patients achieved the same clinical results whether you increased the steroid dose or added a long-acting beta-agonist, sometimes the latter did even better.

Now if there is indeed a carry-over effect by steroids in the one group of patients, and a lack of symptomatic relief with increased inhaled steroids in the other, contrasting maybe with the relieving effect of long-acting beta-agonists – particularly of those with fast onset –, then, taking all together, I speculate that the compliance with the long-acting beta-agonists will be better than the one with inhaled steroids. Now we are left with a question: Should we do a prospective study comparing these two? You know that the Americans have such a multicenter study under way, sponsored by the NIH. If we respect the positive role of the better compliance, then we have to look at the clinical outcomes!

Dr. Kummer: I feel, philosophy sometimes gives the right direction, but then we should try to get our feet back down on the solid ground. And my question is, can we do so by inventing reliable, non-invasive measures to assess the degree of inflammation? Because what we are talking about is, are we indeed treating the patient well? In the short run, yes, but in the long run? Is it good for the patient to manage his own step down until nil therapy and remain well? Maybe twenty years later, he will come down with severely inflammatory type of COPD and bronchial obstruction. We don't know. So what measures, in your opinion, do we have in the future, which can be made sensitive enough to pick up the degree and dynamics of inflammation without doing biopsies?

Dr. Fabbri: Obviously, this is induced sputum and nitric oxide. But sputum needs a lot of work. It's very variable, and we are working on that. And I don't know whether we will ever reach an intra-subject variability low enough to be able to design it as a clinical tool. The other is nitric oxide, which still is a matter of investigation. Doing biopsies is considered the gold standard. But at the present time, I don't think we have enough evidence to show that the pathology predicts clinical outcome. So I don't know. Of course, research has to go on. And I'd like to have the opinion of the people in the audience whether we do need to measure the pathology to assess the effects. We don't have a Framingham study for the asthmatics. So we don't know what happens with time. We don't know whether they live shorter. Some data suggest that they die earlier. But who is the subject who dies we don't know. We don't know whether severe asthma is just a different disease. It's an open question.

To answer your question, I think that the most direct, most promising, non-invasive would be the nitric oxide and particularly the sputum. Regarding the other sophisticated markers, I think that there is very little evidence that these are more than counting the number of eosinophils.

Dr. Kummer: So that means we should go ahead and standardise the methods for induced sputum production?

Dr. Fabbri: There are several groups working on this subject. There are two methods, and we are trying to combine the two, and probably we will have a tool in the laboratory pretty soon. It's slightly difficult to get the sample, and the procedure itself is potentially dangerous. It's non-invasive, because you don't put anything through the mouth or through the nose. But you give an aerosol of hypertonic saline. And I described death in a subject who underwent an inhalation challenge with distilled water. So I wouldn't be surprised that something like that happens with nebulized hypertonic saline. So I think it is non-invasive, but that doesn't mean that it is not risky. With the nitric oxide I don't see any problem of this kind.

Dr. Boyd: I just think that we are committed to these lines of approach to clinical research and that we must examine the histology and the evolution of these inflammatory responses that have been described. I think, as clinicians, we're going to have to wait until this information becomes available. I just believe that our patients are still dictating how the therapy is used and how the balance of the management will work out. But I think the clinician also has to be entrepreneurial and listen to the speakers from yesterday who're looking at basic mechanisms. One of the things which I thought was fascinating yesterday was the possible link with infection and the microbiologist's contribution to changes within the airways, that relate to infection, that appear to be modulated by therapy. So I think the clinician has to be a bit of everything, including a bit patient.

Dr. Fabbri: Nowadays, the gastroenterologists call the gastric ulcer just an infectious disease. We might do the same in a few years, with asthma!

Dr. Boyd: Maybe there's nothing new under the sun and by maintaining an open mind and a broad view, we can look at possible links that may open up new areas that are just as valid.

Dr. Fabbri: Thank you for this stimulating discussion.

SpringerMedizin

Friedrich Kummer (Hrsg.)

Asthma

Structural Basis – Theophylline Today
Strukturelle Grundlagen – Theophyllin heute

1995. 37 Abbildungen. X, 197 Seiten.
Broschiert DM 66,–, öS 462,–. ISBN 3-211-82670-X

Die strukturellen Veränderungen der Bronchialschleimhaut beim Asthma sind zwar Folge der zellulären Interaktionen, aber wesentlich träger als diese und bilden die Basis für später irreversible Funktionsstörungen. Daher ist die frühe antientzündliche Therapie so wichtig. Für diese wieder scheint das Theophyllin zunehmend interessant zu werden, wie aus neuesten in vitro und in vivo Untersuchungen hervorgeht.

The structural changes of the bronchial mucosa in asthma are consequences of cellular interactions. They appear more sluggish than the latter, and they form the basis for the irreversible component of the functional disorder. This underlines the importance of early antiinflammatory treatment. In this context, our interest in theophyllin as a modulator of inflammation has been evoked recently, supported by the latest in vitro and in vivo results.

SpringerWienNewYork

Sachsenplatz 4-6, P.O.Box 89, A-1201 Wien, Fax +43-1-330 24 26,
e-mail: order@springer.at, Internet: http://www.springer.at
New York, NY 10010, 175 Fifth Avenue • D-14197 Berlin, Heidelberger Platz 3
Tokyo 113, 3-13, Hongo 3-chome, Bunkyo-ku

SpringerMedizin

Friedrich Kummer (Hrsg.)

Asthma

Immunopathology and Immunotherapy
Immunopathologie und Immunotherapie

1993. 33 Abbildungen. XII, 179 Seiten.
Broschiert DM 59,–, öS 415,–. ISBN 3-211-82454-5

Das Konzept des allergischen Asthma hat lange Zeit so sehr dominiert, daß die Immunotherapie vielfach ohne gesicherte diagnostische Grundlage, halbherzig oder ohne die Feinheiten der Allergenvermeidung angewendet wurde. Die Forschung der letzten zehn Jahre hat uns eine derartige Ausweitung unseres Wissenshorizontes beschert, daß es an der Zeit schien, maßgebliche Autoren zur gemeinsamen Diskussion der neuen Aspekte einzuladen. Das Buch berichtet von den neuesten Erkenntnissen über zelluläres Verhalten, unterschiedliche Zytokinmuster und autoimmunologische Aspekte bis hin zur modernen Allergenvermeidung, aber auch von der wirksamen medikamentösen Therapie der eosinophilen Entzündung

The concept of asthma being an "allergic disorder only" has dominated above others to an extent, that a re-evaluation of this issue in the light of very recent results from research in immunopathology seemed more than overdue.
This volume provides a current concept of theory and clinical practice of immunopathology and therapy of asthma, comprising extensive and brand new laboratory data on atopy, intrinsic asthma, aspects of autoimmunology, as well as guidelines for allergen avoidance, immunotherapy and – last not least – pharmacological treatment of eosinophilic inflammation.

SpringerWienNewYork

Sachsenplatz 4-6, P.O.Box 89, A-1201 Wien, Fax +43-1-330 24 26,
e-mail: order@springer.at, Internet: http://www.springer.at
New York, NY 10010, 175 Fifth Avenue • D-14197 Berlin, Heidelberger Platz 3
Tokyo 113, 3-13, Hongo 3-chome, Bunkyo-ku

Springer-Verlag
and the Environment

WE AT SPRINGER-VERLAG FIRMLY BELIEVE THAT AN international science publisher has a special obligation to the environment, and our corporate policies consistently reflect this conviction.

WE ALSO EXPECT OUR BUSINESS PARTNERS – PRINTERS, paper mills, packaging manufacturers, etc. – to commit themselves to using environmentally friendly materials and production processes.

THE PAPER IN THIS BOOK IS MADE FROM NO-CHLORINE pulp and is acid free, in conformance with international standards for paper permanency.

GPSR Compliance

The European Union's (EU) General Product Safety Regulation (GPSR) is a set of rules that requires consumer products to be safe and our obligations to ensure this.

If you have any concerns about our products, you can contact us on ProductSafety@springernature.com

In case Publisher is established outside the EU, the EU authorized representative is:

Springer Nature Customer Service Center GmbH
Europaplatz 3
69115 Heidelberg, Germany

Batch number: 10577917

Printed by Printforce, the Netherlands